Sandra Hempel is a journalist and copywriter who specializes in health and social issues. She has worked for many leading newspapers and magazines, including the *Times*, *Sunday Times*, *Guardian* and *Mail on Sunday*, as well as for the Department of Health and the NHS. She lives in London with her two daughters.

THE
MEDICAL DETECTIVE

John Snow, Cholera and the Mystery
of the Broad Street Pump

SANDRA HEMPEL

Granta Books
London

Granta Publications, 12 Addison Avenue, London W11 4QR

First published in Great Britain by Granta Books, 2006
This edition published by Granta Books, 2007

A CIP catalogue record for this book is available
from the British Library.

3 5 7 9 10 8 6 4 2

Typeset by M Rules
Printed in the UK by CPI Bookmarque, Croydon, CR0 4TD

CONTENTS

ACKNOWLEDGEMENTS

An enormous thank-you to Dr David Gardner-Medwin of Newcastle upon Tyne, who originally agreed to read an early chapter of *The Medical Detective*, but then generously allowed himself to be persuaded to read the entire manuscript, section by section, as I wrote it. His depth of learning in both history and medicine as well as his wide general knowledge were invaluable, as were his suggestions and encouragement throughout the writing process.

Thanks also to Andrew Cunningham, Wellcome Trust senior research fellow in the history of medicine, University of Cambridge, and to Dr Peter Tiplady, director of public health, North Cumbria (retired), both of whom read the entire draft, corrected errors and boosted my morale with their enthusiasm. Friend Dr Mike Smith, MBBS, DPH, MFPHM, Dobst RCOG, specialist in preventative medicine and medical communicator, read chapters, gave excellent advice and has been a fantastic source of encouragement and support.

Professor Nigel Paneth of Michigan State University; Professor David A. Sack, International Centre for Diarrhoeal Disease Research, Centre for Health and Population Research, Dhaka, Bangladesh, and Professor, Department of International Health, Johns Hopkins University; Professor John Hamilton, Professor Emeritus, Durham University, UK, and Dr Denis Smith, PhD, MSc, DIC, C.Eng, engineering historian, were all approached completely out of the blue and immediately offered to help. They read relevant chapters and freely gave me the benefit of their vast knowledge as well as their support. Dr Milton Wainwright, senior lecturer, Department of Molecular Biology and Biotechnology, University of Sheffield, shared his work on the history of microbiology with me, including papers still in press.

Thanks for advice and support to friends Jane Seymour, MSc, and Jeremy Preston, one of the world's great librarians. Thanks also to Peter Goddard, FRCPath, honorary librarian, Royal College of Pathologists, and to the Royal Society of Chemistry for dealing with queries.

My brilliant agent, Patrick Walsh, steered me with cheerful and practised skill through the tricky business of turning an idea and a couple of sketchy chapters into a professional proposal. My editor at Granta, Sara Holloway, kept the lightest yet surest touch on the work and was a joy to work with. I was very lucky in that both she and Colette Vella were so in tune with my ideas. Wendy Moore, author of *The Knife Man*, provided essential moral support throughout.

And finally thanks to my daughters, the amazing Georgia and Sophie, mainly for just being around, but also for putting up with me for the last couple of years without once resorting to violence. My beloved husband Bob Nibbs, who died in 2004, encouraged me from the start, as he did in anything I have ever tried to achieve – and still does.

Sandra Hempel, 2005

To my beloved husband
Bob Nibbs, 1947–2004
Until I see you again

On the floor before the fireplace extended on a palliasse, covered with a solitary blanket and surrounded by a group of female friends, lay a girl of slender make and juvenile height but with the face of a superannuated hag. She uttered no moan but languidly flung herself from side to side and from the supine to the prone position. The colour of her countenance was that of lead – a silver blue, ghastly tint; her eyes were sunk deep in their sockets as though they had been driven in an inch behind their natural position; her mouth was squared; her eyelids black; her fingers shrunk, bent and inky in their hue. All pulse was gone at the wrist and a tenacious sweat moistened her bosom. In short, Sir, that face and form I can never forget, were I to live beyond the period of a man's natural age.

. . . Would to God I could bring the sceptics here. And if they can confound the exhaustion consequent on the vomiting and purging of English cholera with the sudden, deadly, overwhelming collapse – the living death – of the unhappy being who will probably have perished before my letter closes . . . I shall forever after follow the philosophy of the man who doubted his own existence.

London physician Dr William O'Shaughnessy describing what
he saw on a visit to Sunderland in the Autumn of 1831

INTRODUCTION

The Long Journey

A malady yet more terrible than the yellow fever appeared on the banks of the Ganges. After having devastated India and desolated Persia, it showed itself at length in Syria and now threatens destruction even amongst European nations

M. Keraudren, *Memoire sur le Cholera Morbus de l'Inde*, 1831

Cholera first stepped out onto the world stage in 1817. No one knows exactly when or how the tiny bacterium responsible for the disease evolved, but its ancestry goes back to the origins of life itself. We do know that it first emerged from the Sunderbund swamps of the Ganges Delta in north-east India where, in all probability, it had been mutating for millennia.

Each disease-causing organism is a threat only to particular species – in all the rest it is impotent – and the *Vibrio cholerae* is particularly discerning, although not unique, in this respect, for it reserves its attack for one species alone, a latecomer to the planet. Only with the arrival of *Homo sapiens* did the *Vibrio cholerae* show itself for the killer that it is.

Cholera has probably been endemic to India for hundreds of years. Ancient Indian texts describe a disease that is almost certainly cholera, and there are accounts by sixteenth-century Portuguese colonists, including the physician Garcia D'Orta, who spent many years in Goa in south-west India. D'Orta refers to what he calls: 'the choleric passion, which the Indians call morxi, or disease from eating too much', before going on to list precisely the symptoms of cholera. There are also some isolated early accounts outside India of what sound like the same disease, although it is impossible to know for sure. In 1629, for example, the Dutch physician Jacob Bontius wrote about 'a terrible disorder' encountered in Batavia, now Jakarta, in Indonesia, that he called cholera, 'which quickly precipitates the wretched sufferer in excruciating agony to the grave'. Only in the early 1800s, however, did accounts began to crop up regularly in medical records, and then only after cholera had had the temerity to threaten Europeans in what were to become three great nineteenth-century pandemics, each of which originated in India.

The disease gets its name from the Greek words for 'bile' – the bitter, brownish fluid secreted by the liver – and 'to flow'; in other words, a flow of bile or bilious disease. In ancient Greek medicine, the term 'cholera' referred to any severe vomiting and diarrhoea, but in the nineteenth century when a specific, mysterious and deadly form of these symptoms began to spread across the world, 'Asian' and 'Indian' cholera and 'cholera morbus' were used to describe it. As the disease approached countries where it was previously unknown, doctors sometimes wrongly diagnosed a case of severe diarrhoea and vomiting as Asian cholera. When the genuine disease appeared, however, such mistakes were usually only too clear.

In the first great pandemic, from 1817–23, cholera spread beyond India into Asia, while in the second, from 1826 until 1837 or so, it moved from Asia into Europe to lay waste the great cities of the developed world. And the third, beginning in 1846, lasted for some twenty years before it, too, dissipated and vanished.

The first official British reports of an epidemic describe an outbreak of a strange and deadly illness in Jessore – the capital of the Sunderbunds in the north-eastern province of Bengal – a crowded, filthy city ravaged by malaria and surrounded by impenetrable jungle. On 28 August 1817, the British government received a report that 'a malignant disorder had broken out attacking all classes of natives promiscuously and destroying from 20 to 30 inhabitants every day. So destructive was it in mortality, so unexplained in character that the inhabitants, astonished and terrified at the unaccountable and very destructive inroads of the pestilence, fled in crowds to the country as the only means of escaping impending death. In the course of a few weeks, 10,000 of the inhabitants perished in this single district.'

This then was a 'shock disease', even at a time and in a part of the world where killer epidemics were common; and the British doctor Ashbel Smith later described some of the cases he had witnessed. Cholera often struck so fast that patients said it was like being hit with a club, he wrote. 'A sudden and great increase of a previous diarrhoea . . . is in most cases the first symptom. Vomiting occurs simultaneously or soon follows . . . [and then] cramps occupying the soles of the feet, the calves of the legs, the thighs and . . . the extremities supervene.'

Just an hour later, Smith said, the sufferer takes on 'that frightful choleric decomposition of the features of which language can convey no adequate idea . . . voice nearly extinct or heard only in a feeble whisper; extremities cold, shrunk, livid or marbled; the skin of the hands, forearms and feet . . . wrinkled like a washerwoman's . . . scrotum livid and contracted . . . thirst torturing . . . From a vein opened, the blood flows not at all or with great difficulty, is of a deep, dark colour, and at the end of some hours resembles a feebly coagulated vegetable jelly.'

Smith described the cramps as atrocious, and another British doctor named Whiting was shocked by his first encounter with severe choleraic cramp. 'I never in my life saw anything equal to it, except in a case of hydrophobia [rabies],' he told his colleagues . . . 'The patient was wracked by the most intense spasms it is possible to conceive, every muscle of the body was in a state of the most plastic [pliable, and here, presumably, mishapen] contraction, the muscles of the abdomen were gathered up into folds and knots, the knees were drawn up to the head, the arms were forcibly bent and the whole frame was writhing in the most dreadful agony, the patient shrieking in a manner truly awful. I tried to get down some laudanum but the attempt was useless.'

On 6 November 1817, it was the turn of the British – the 'malignant disorder' struck the Grand Army commanded by the Marquis of Hastings and stationed in Bundelkhand in central India, where the British government had just signed a treaty acquiring all rights over the territory. The death toll was an astonishing 9,000 men, 5,000 of whom died in five days alone. 'The invasion was so sudden and violent that the horsemen were stricken from their steeds and in vain attempted to remount; and the roads were covered with the dying and the dead,' wrote the Marquis. In its severest form, cholera is one of the most rapidly fatal illnesses known to man, and a previously healthy person can die in two or three hours.

From Bundelkhand, the disease soon spread to the whole Indian peninsula, from where it was carried by British troops into Nepal, Afghanistan and Muscat (Oman). And it still had a long way to go. Before this first pandemic was over, it was to stretch east into Mauritius, Thailand, Burma, Sumatra, Java, Borneo, the Philippines, China, Japan and south into parts of Africa.

Some dramatic accounts of its progress through the Middle East come from a British traveller named James Fraser who, in 1821, made a great journey through the region. By the time the disease reached Bendar Abassi in modern Iran, where one-sixth of the population died, the picture had become a familiar one: the bazaars closed, houses abandoned, dead bodies heaped in the streets and a mass exodus of everyone still able to run.

By September 1821 – almost four years after it had massacred British troops at Bundelkhand – the mystery sickness had reached Shiraz in south-central Iran, choosing the Prince Royal's harem as one of its first targets and carrying off the British consul, a notable amateur scientist called Rich. Here the locals tried a novel means of trying to frighten off the invader, as Fraser described:

Salvos of artillery and peals of musketry roared from the rising to the setting sun, loud shouts were raised by united thousands, and gongs and trumpets increased the horrid commotion, but the unrelenting progress of the pestilence soon allowed the inefficacy of this clamour, and the crash of ordnance and martial music gave place to the shrieks and melancholy wailings of the dying and the bereaved.

After a winter lull, the disease re-emerged in Iran to strike towns along the caravan routes which led north-west from Ispaham. From there it moved into Armenia, then reaching Erzurum in eastern Turkey just as the Persian prince, Abbas Mirza, busy fighting the Turks, had managed to surround his enemy. But the conqueror's army was soon attacked by a stronger force: 'The cholera swept his ranks from front to rear and his terror-stricken soldiers threw down their arms in dismay and fled before this invisible destroyer.'

That Teheran managed to escape an outbreak greatly interested those trying to fathom this unpredictable malady's ways. A caravan had been travelling the country at the time from south to north and its arrival at each town on its route appeared to coincide with an outbreak of the disease. When the merchants approached the Shah's palace in Teheran then, they received a Royal Proclamation forbidding them to come any closer, so they turned aside in a wide detour, leaving Teheran untouched by cholera. Again though, it was noted, outbreaks continued to dog the caravan on its new itinerary.

Modern Iraq suffered even worse than Iran. In Basra, one-third of the population – 18,000 people – died in just eleven days, before Baghdad succumbed and also lost a third of its population. In July 1822, the disease appeared in Mosul, sixty miles north of Baghdad, before heading west into Syria where, the following June, Latakia and Antioch were infected and then the capital Damascus. The port of Latakia in north-west Syria, which was badly hit, lies on a promontory projecting into the Mediterranean, a short sea voyage away from Europe. In five years, the disease had killed hundreds of thousands as it travelled some 4,500 miles from its origins in the Sunderbunds swamp-waters. Yet, for reasons that no one could fathom, the Europeans had escaped.

But hardly had this first pandemic died than the second began, three years later in 1826. Again, the source was the Ganges Delta and again the disease spread quickly across the Indian subcontinent. This time it travelled further, and was eventually to kill millions from the United States to North Africa and Cuba. Such was the scale of this outbreak that 30,000 people in Cairo and Alexandria are said to have died in one twenty-four-hour period alone.

The first American victims were an Irish immigrant family called Fitzgerald living in New York. Fitzgerald himself was the first to fall sick, coming home late one night with violent stomach pains, but by the time the doctor arrived the next morning, he had recovered. His wife and children were not to be so lucky, however, and within two days they were dead. Quickly, the disease spread throughout the city, killing hundreds, mainly among the poor, but terrifying all New Yorkers alike. 'The roads in all directions were lined with well-filled stage coaches fleeing from the city, as we may suppose the inhabitants of Pompei fled when the red lava showered down on their houses,' wrote one eye-witness. From New York, cholera fanned out over most of the country, hitting nearly all of the major cities, before it finally petered out two years later. Five thousand people died in New Orleans alone.

Fear travelled hand-in-hand with cholera, and the Philippines was the scene of a particular panic. 'In the Philippine Islands, the malady was marked by one of those terrific outbursts of barbarian despair which have more than once signalised the progress of this pestilence,' wrote an observer. 'The Chinese and Europeans were accused of magic by the superstitious crowd and numbers of them were massacred on the shore within sight of an English vessel.' Among those to be stabbed, beaten and left for dead was a French naturalist called Godfroi 'whose collection of reptiles and insects lent especial countenance to their insane accusations'.

In 1827, a year after the second pandemic began, cholera crossed from Afghanistan to Bukhara in Russia. By the summer of 1829, it was in Orenburg at the southern tip of the Urals. Within its sights were Moscow and then, unthinkably, St Petersburg, the glittering capital of the Russian empire. This time, Europe trembled.

CHAPTER 1

A Country Holds its Breath

If it be really true that there is a 'pestilence which walketh in darkness', observing no regular or even track, desolating various parts of Europe simultaneously, pursuing its murderous course in the face of adverse winds and visiting countries in which it had never before been heard of, who can say that England will be exempt?

H. K. Randell, London surgeon, September 1831

On 15 September 1830, Lord Heytesbury, His Majesty's Ambassador Extraordinary and Plenipotentiary to the Emperor of all the Russias, wrote to the Right Hon. the Earl of Aberdeen, KT, His Majesty's Secretary of State for Foreign Affairs in London:

My Lord,

The accounts of the progress of the cholera morbus are now becoming rather alarming. It is making rapid advances towards Moscow; it is already at Sinebiask, Tyaritzigur, Saretaff and Pewza. At Astrakhan, the governor, his son, and almost every officer of police have perished and the other deaths are at the rate of about 100 daily. If the disease once reaches Moscow there can be little doubt that it will spread to St Petersburg, Warsaw and thence into Germany.

This will be much less extraordinary than its regular progress from India into the southern provinces of the Russian empire.

It appears to be of a very deadly nature and to have all the
character of the real Indian cholera.

I have the honour to be, &c

Heytesbury

The situation was, in fact, much worse than Heytesbury had
described, for even as the ink dried on the diplomat's letter,
Moscow had fallen. Nor had His Excellency exaggerated the
tragedy that had been played out at Astrakhan earlier that summer:
the great trading city of the Volga delta, some 900 miles south-east
of Moscow, had been decimated. The whole bustling commercial
centre ground to a halt. The bank suspended operations, the
bazaars fell silent and even the bars stood empty. With a deathly
quiet hanging over the city, the only signs of life came from the
constant stream of funeral processions; and as the mourners
wound their way through the streets, they passed the bodies of
those who had fallen as they tried to run, rotting at the roadsides.
The grave-diggers, unequal to their grisly task, threw up their
hands in defeat and tossed a thousand corpses into one hastily dug
sand-pit.

Terrifying as this new disease was, it had not much concerned
the 'civilised' world so long as it confined itself to exotic countries
such as India and Persia, but once it crossed the psychological and
geographic divide from Asiatic into European Russia, the unimag-
inable had happened. As Lord Heytesbury had predicted, with
Moscow now hit, cholera was heading straight for the great Tsarist
capital of St Petersburg.

His Excellency, William à Court, 1st Baron Heytesbury, was not
the only member of King William IV's foreign service to be informing London about the journey of the *cholera morbus*. From consuls
and embassies throughout Eastern, Central and Northern Europe,
British diplomats were tracking its progress as it edged towards
them. Two days after Heytesbury had voiced his concerns, James
Yeames, at the British consulate in Odessa, the Black Sea port 700
miles south of St Petersburg, was passing on the grim news from

his brother in south-west Russia that the disease had just struck at Cherkassy in the Ukraine. 'The acting Governor-General proceeded from hence three days ago to the infected districts, and troops have been assembled for the formation of cordons,' Yeames told the ambassador. 'A sanitary line has been already formed at a short distance from Taganrog, a precaution in which much confidence does not seem to be placed,' he added, ending with the gloomy reflection: 'The cholera morbus, observed since some years to be traversing all Asia in a direction towards Europe, is thus already at our door.'

Three weeks later, the disease was finally officially confirmed in Moscow, and so, on 9 October, Tsar Nicholas, Emperor of all the Russias, set out on the 460-mile journey from St Petersburg to lift the spirits of the Muscovites, accompanied only by his doctor and a single aide-de-camp. By now, the situation in Russia was so bad that Lord Heytesbury feared for the peace of the continent. As he saw it, if this sickness left one of the main pillars of the balance of power no longer able to muster a fighting force, then the stability of all Europe was threatened.

> The present state of Russia cannot be contemplated without fear and dismay [he told the Foreign Secretary]. All the country extending from Tiflis [now Tiblisi, capital of Georgia], Astrakan and Orenburg to Moscow is devastated by a pestilence which may probably ere long spread over the rest of the empire . . . All communication and all commerce are suspended and all recruiting for the army becomes impossible. The lately victorious army of Bulgaria exists no longer but in name. Nothing but skeleton regiments have come back from the Turkish war. Russia may almost be considered hors-de-combat for the moment.

Tsar Nicholas in the meantime, with an impressive energy and lack of concern for his own well-being, had set about visiting every hospital in Moscow, but even His Imperial Majesty The Emperor of all the Russias could do nothing to stem the force of the catastrophe now

unleashed upon the city. By the end of October, with no official figures available, the most reliable sources were putting the total number
of cholera cases among the total population of 300,000 at 2,500,
with 1,100 dead and hopes fading fast for most of the rest of the
infected. Three weeks later, the number of cases hovered at just under
5,000 and the death toll stood at 2,660.

In Britain in December, Ambassador Heytesbury's master, Lord
Aberdeen, was replaced as Foreign Secretary by the formidable
Lord Palmerston, who lost no time at all in turning his attention to
the threat from the East. Heytesbury was told to find an eminent
physician from among the British community in St Petersburg and
send him off to Moscow without delay to study the disease and
report back to London. A Dr Thomas Walker declared himself
ready to take on the task for £5 a day plus expenses and, as the
Foreign Secretary had given Heytesbury no idea of how much he
was allowed to pay, the diplomat quickly accepted the doctor's
terms. 'I have been obliged to use my own discretion in fixing it,' he
wrote, adding that if Palmerston disagreed, Dr Walker could easily
be recalled. However, as the physician was giving up a lucrative
practice in St Petersburg and taking a considerable personal risk,
the ambassador said he saw nothing extravagant in Walker's
demands. Nor, it seemed, did the British government, and Dr
Walker duly packed his bags and, like Tsar Nicholas before him,
set off for the cholera hospitals of Moscow.

By April 1831, there was more bad news. James Yeames reported
from Odessa that the disease was now edging worryingly close to
the Polish border. Conveniently, in this corner of the Russian empire
there existed a despised minority who could be blamed for this
latest disaster. With the appalling anti-Semitism of his day, then perfectly acceptable in the politest of circles, Heytesbury noted cholera's
arrival among the Jewish community in Podolia in the Ukraine,
commenting: 'The Jews, filthy and gregarious as they are, will soon
convey the disease into Volhynia and thence into Poland.' Quite
whom he considered responsible for the disease's previous advance
across land and water, respecting no borders, His Excellency did not

explain. In fact, while cholera did indeed quickly make its way into Poland, some of the first reports came from the fortress of Zamosc on the banks of the River Labunka, where a detachment of Russian soldiers had been ordered in to suppress an uprising. Soon the disease had spread from the Russian to the Polish army, and it then made its way steadily westwards through towns and villages, to Danzig and right into the heart of the capital Warsaw.

At the end of May, Thomas Tupper, His Majesty's consul in the Latvian port of Riga on the Baltic, was writing to tell Heytesbury of sixty deaths from cholera in that city, including the masters of four British merchant ships and several crew members. The disease was thus moving north as well as west, and was now a mere 140 miles from St Petersburg. In a half-hearted attempt to stop it reaching the Russian capital, the authorities set up a quarantine for all goods and travellers from Riga by sea and by land, only to relax it almost at once for fear of frightening the public and disrupting trade.

Before June was out, the inevitable had happened. On the 28th of that month, it became the ambassador's sad duty to inform Lord Palmerston that two cases of cholera had been diagnosed in St Petersburg. Both of the victims were boatmen who worked on the waterways, transporting goods from the interior to the capital. The news was greeted almost immediately by riots in the streets. As the disease began to spread, the authorities started forcibly removing not only the sick, but those who were merely old, infirm or drunk. Rumours ran through the city: all those taken to hospital were being poisoned and their bodies used for dissection; all those taken to hospital were being poisoned and their bodies used in black magic rituals; the disease had been invented by the doctors and police in order to extort money from the people; the sick were being buried alive. Angry mobs began attacking hospitals in order to 'liberate' the sick and dying, beating and killing doctors in the process, while groups of vigilantes prowled the streets, searching for suspicious-looking characters upon whom to vent their fear and fury. Several people unfortunate enough to be discovered with bottles of quack remedies about their persons were denounced as poisoners and beaten to death on the spot.

Three days after cholera struck the Russian capital, the British doctor David Barry arrived with his colleague William Russell. The pair had been on their way to Riga to study the disease there but, learning that quarantines had been set up on their intended route and that, in any case, the subject of their quest had advanced to meet them, they decided to break their journey in St Petersburg. Barry found himself caught up in a nightmare of what to him were the strange, unwholesome customs of the people and of this sickness that left its victims whining like dogs, he said, their black-purple, still-living bodies already resembling the corpses that they were soon to become. And as if further misery were needed, the doctors found St Petersburg in the middle of a heatwave, fanned by burning winds from the East. The temperature in their airless apartment seldom dipped below eighty degrees. Barry reported:

> The sufferings . . . have furnished me with the type of disease which I had certainly never seen before, which cannot be forgotten after having been observed nor, I think, confounded with any other malady. The people are in the midst of a solemn fast, the streets thronged with processions and other more tumultuous meetings, the churches are filled all day. Many are attacked after coming from these meetings and some have suffered while attending them. The coarse, acescent [sour, acidic] food; the sheepskin clothing of the peasants, seldom changed and worn even at this season; the protracted religious fasts; the subsequent intemperance, both in eating and drinking; the intolerably close apartments of Russians of all ranks; the consequent sensibility to sudden change of temperature, render them . . . particularly liable to suffering.

Barry's colleague Dr Russell, who unlike Barry had had wide experience of cholera with the army in India, suggested that the pair take charge of some of the patients in one of the military hospitals, an offer that the hard-pressed medical authorities accepted gratefully until the danger from the mob made Barry and Russell think again. 'The violent excitement of the people . . . more particularly against medical men whom they lately looked upon as emissaries employed by their enemies to poison them, has rendered our proposition inadmissable,' Barry explained. An uneasy peace was restored when Tsar Nicholas, now back in residence at his great estate of Peterhoff, appeared in the Hay Market to confront his unruly subjects: 'Are you Poles or French, to act so?' he reportedly thundered, reminding them that the doctors were risking their own lives in trying to save theirs.

Barry marvelled at what he saw as the Emperor's almost magical powers: 'This city is now tranquil and the poor, deluded people beg for the assistance of the very men whom but a day or two ago they would have torn to pieces,' he noted in astonishment. The rather less impressionable Heytesbury, however, thought that this new calm owed rather more to the sheer intensity of the disease. 'Where 600 are falling ill daily, it is difficult to be sceptical upon the subject,' the ambassador observed.

Despite the months of warning, cholera's final arrival in the capital had still found St Petersburg totally unprepared. There were not nearly enough hospitals to accommodate the sick nor doctors to staff them. Some of the victims were carted about the streets from hospital to hospital, being refused admittance everywhere, only to die in the road. Most of the government fled the city as soon as the first cases appeared, and even the Emperor had now retreated behind an impenetrable cordon around his palace. And then there was the usual difficulty in Tsarist Russia of obtaining accurate information on any subject of any importance whatsoever. Dr Walker, the physician employed by Ambassador Heytesbury, was now in St Petersburg and trying to compile his report for the British government, but was unable to get hold of the basic facts and figures. When Sir James McGregor, the Director General of Army Hospitals in London, sent him some urgent queries, Walker made his frustrations clear: 'From the anxiety expressed in your letter which I received last night, I hasten to reply, although it is merely to say that I have nothing worthwhile to say,' he wrote, adding: 'You can have no idea of the difficulty of getting the truth here without [unless] you know the country – the Medical Council of the Empire have not themselves got proper reports.'

In August 1831, the Russians gave up trying to impose cordons around the infected areas in their vast land. Their attempts had long descended into farce anyway. All restrictions were removed with the exception of those around the imperial palace – now it would be seen once and for all whether quarantine worked, Heytesbury remarked – leaving the disease officially free to run where it would throughout the empire. At the same time, the authorities finally released the casualty figures for St Petersburg: in five weeks, over 10,000 out of a population of 440,000 people had died.

That summer, as the death toll shot up across Europe, the British government, determined to be better prepared than their shambolic Russian counterparts, had been doing more than simply shuddering over the despatches now thudding on to desks at the Foreign Office from all over the Continent. When King William IV opened a new session of Parliament on 21 June 1831, he told his audience: 'It is with deep concern that I have to announce to you the continued progress of this formidable disease in the Eastern parts of Europe.'

The first real note of concern in the country had been sounded the previous October when the government released the text of Ambassador Heytesbury's letter, along with a statement from the Privy Council calling for 'the utmost care and vigilance' to be used in dealing with ships arriving from suspect foreign ports, but at that time there had been little public response. Since 1828 the newspapers had carried the occasional small paragraph about cholera, merely noting the progress of the disease, first in India and then in Russia and Poland, but there had been no suggestion that Britain had anything to worry about.

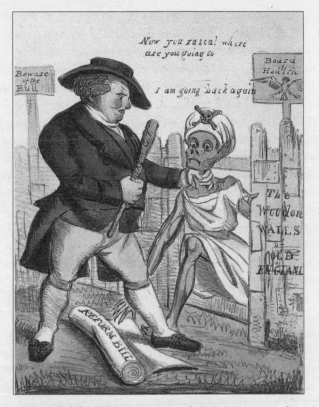

John Bull defending Britain against cholera: resistance to the
1832 Reform Bill satirised

Even now not all of His Majesty's subjects took his warning
seriously. Cynics believed they could detect some government
spin-doctoring in these tales of death and destruction: after all, the
cholera panic had arrived just in time to divert attention away from
the controversial Reform Bill whose passage through Parliament
was threatening to cause riots in the streets. Others blamed an
irresponsible media. The prominent London physician Dr James
Johnson wrote furiously to *The Times* to accuse the paper of whipping up 'that terrible malady, cholera-phobia' that was 'raging
like an epidemic throughout the British Isles'. 'The cholera-phobia

will frighten to death a far greater number of Britons than the monster itself will ever destroy by his actual presence,' Johnson wrote. The doctor was soon to be proven very wrong.

The government's first step was to set up a Board of Health to advise it on what action to take. This had been done once before, in 1805, when the country was worried about the threat of a fever from Spain. The new Board was to meet every day under the illustrious control of Sir Henry Halford, President of the Royal College of Physicians and consultant to George III, George IV and now William IV. The *Lancet*, questioning Sir Henry's suitability for his new role, largely on the grounds that he knew nothing about *cholera morbus*, conceded that the knight 'may be well qualified to instruct us on how to endure the noxious atmosphere of a court'.

Sir Henry's services to royalty even extended to monarchs who were long dead. In 1813 he had been at Windsor Castle in the presence of the then Prince of Wales, later George IV, for the opening of what was believed to be the coffin of Charles I. In order to identify the body, Sir Henry had inspected the executed king's severed head. 'On holding up the head to examine the place of separation from the body . . . the fourth cervical vertebra was found to be cut through its substance transversely, leaving the surface of the divided portions perfectly smooth and even, an appearance which could have been produced only by a heavy blow inflicted with a very sharp instrument,' he wrote. Sir Henry would eventually go on to add Queen Victoria to his list of patients before his career in medicine and social climbing was done.

Assisting Sir Henry was a formidable body of the great and the good: The Honourable Edward Stewart, Deputy Chairman of the Board of Customs; Sir Thomas Byam Martin, Comptroller of His Majesty's Navy; Sir William Burnett, Commissioner of the Victualling Office; Sir James McGregor, Director General of Army Hospitals and Sir William Pym, Superintendent General of Quarantine, along with a group of Fellows of Sir Henry's Royal College. On 21 June, while the King was opening Parliament, the Board duly assembled at the headquarters of the Royal College of Physicians in London's Pall

Mall East, one of the most fashionable parts of town, and listened carefully as Sir Henry read out their instructions from the Lords of His Majesty's Most Honourable Privy Council.

They had a considerable task on their hands. They were to look at the existing quarantine regulations and advise their Lordships as and when changes were needed. They must study reports from people like Dr Walker about the disease in Russia and write some guidance about prevention and treatment. They were to draw up rules and regulations for magistrates, doctors and other interested parties about how to contain a local outbreak. And in particular, their Lordships asked the Board to 'give their attention to the points which are the most important in this enquiry: whether this disease is communicable from person to person and whether it is communicable by inanimate matter of any description'. It was the big question and until it was settled beyond all doubt, no government could be certain that it was taking the right action to protect its people. Sir Henry and his colleagues were urged to 'examine any persons who may be able to throw any light upon these points', which hinted at just how deeply in the dark about the matter were their Lordships of the Privy Council, the members of the Royal College of Physicians, Sir Henry Halford and everyone else in the country.

The immediate priority, however, the Privy Council said, was to advise on how long travellers from infected ports should be held in quarantine, which types of imported goods were most likely to carry the disease and what were the best methods of disinfection. They were told to make a start by looking at the ideas of a certain Dr Ure, who suggested fumigating cargoes by pouring chlorine gas down tubes into ships' holds – a method, Ure insisted, that was cheap, effective and, very importantly, guaranteed to do no harm to the goods. 'After 24 hours the hatches should be opened and the air round the tubes renewed by free ventilation, during which process the dress and persons of the crew will be sufficiently purified by the diluted chlorine,' he explained, adding that the cargo could then be unloaded with perfect safety, 'for chlorine gas . . . will pervade the substance of every package, having imported its very peculiar, though fleeting, odour to the flocks of wool in the heart of the hardest bale'.

All that was required, Ure believed, was a simple tank in which to produce the gas, a few pipes down which the gas could pass into the hold, and another pipe mounted upright on the deck to allow the existing air in the hold to escape. 'The quantity requisite for destroying any contagion, however virulent, is too small to produce any change in the animal and vegetable fibres of the goods or occasion any expense of more than £10 for purifying the largest ship in the Baltic fleet,' the doctor declared. A sketch of the equipment accompanied his report. The Privy Council was clearly impressed by Dr Ure – so much so that when Sir Henry and his friends, after watching demonstrations on bales of flax, pronounced the process to be impractical, Sir Henry was told by their Lordships to think again. Just days later, then, Dr Ure was to be found at His Majesty's Dockyard, Woolwich, testing out his contraption on a ship under quarantine there, while his colleague, Dr Fincham, was at Chatham, measuring how far chlorine gas could penetrate a given weight of tightly packed hemp.

Now somewhat more enthused about the possibilities of chlorine, the Board of Health went on to sanction some rather strange new experiments, not on bales of rope and cotton this time but on human beings. The research was based on the principle of inoculation introduced into Britain in the 1740s by Lady Mary Wortley Montague, by which an individual was given a mild dose of smallpox using fluid from the pustules of smallpox patients in order to stimulate their body's defences and protect against further attacks. By 1831 this form of smallpox inoculation had been replaced by Edward Jenner's safer practice of vaccination, using fluid from cowpox pustules. While everyone knew that vaccination worked, no one, including Jenner, understood why.

For the purposes of this experiment, people were to be inoculated with some infectious matter that had first been treated with chlorine gas. If they failed to develop the infection, this would prove that the gas had neutralised the disease, the Board reasoned. To do this, the researchers went back to the old pre-Jenner practice, taking fluid from the pustules of patients in a smallpox hospital. One sample was put into a bottle containing one part chlorine gas to twenty-four parts air and another into a bottle containing one part chlorine gas to fifty parts air. After three hours, the samples were removed and three people, one of them a child, were inoculated with the first specimen. In the child's case, the doctors made three scratches in his arm, deep enough to make them bleed profusely, and then stuck a piece of cloth soaked in the smallpox pus over his wounds. Four others, all adults, were inoculated with the second sample which had been exposed to the weaker gas. None of the seven went down with smallpox.

Some time later they were all inoculated again but this time with normal smallpox pus and this time they all developed the disease 'in a perfectly normal manner', said the *Lancet*, although the journal does not record if they all recovered 'in a perfectly normal manner'. The experiment was said to prove that their non-reaction to the first inoculation was due to the gas, rather than to any natural immunity to smallpox, but despite such seemingly promising results, the exercise was condemned as flawed and useless. One error, it was claimed, was that in the first round of inoculations, a third 'control' group of people should have been inoculated with a sample exposed to air alone, in case air was the disinfecting agent. The ethical considerations of using a child in such an exercise seem not to have worried anyone unduly.

As Ure and Fincham busied themselves in the dockyards, and as clinical tests with smallpox pus were underway, the news that the Government had set up a Board of Health was being received with great interest throughout the country. Now, the public appeared to be taking notice. Countless numbers of His Majesty's subjects, it seemed, had expert advice to impart on the subject of the *cholera morbus*. Pouring in by every post came prescriptions for treatments that had never been known to fail, descriptions of remedies that guaranteed protection, and instructions on establishing fail-safe *cordons sanitaires*. One correspondent knew for certain that in cases of cholera, bleeding was the key to recovery, while another had incontrovertible evidence that bleeding hastened the end. Accounts of personal experience that proved beyond doubt that cholera was contagious were matched only by accounts of personal experience that proved beyond doubt that it was not. Medical men with genuine knowledge of the disease, housewives with herbal recipes, quack-remedy salesmen, well-meaning cranks and those with an eye to a well-paid government post: all wanted their say.

A Mr Power of Northampton, for example, had read about the Board in the *London Gazette* and begged leave to offer his services as an inspector of quarantine in any part of the UK. He had spent many years in the East Indies and the Philippine Islands, he explained, was conversant with the Spanish language and could give the most unexceptionable references as to his character and conduct from gentlemen holding official situations. The Board thanked Mr Power and said they would let him know.

They reacted more enthusiastically to a letter from Silas Blandford, Esq., of Piccadilly. Mr Blandford was a retired naval surgeon who had spent many years in India, he told them, during which time he had had hundreds of cholera patients under his care and scarcely lost a single one. 'If tomorrow I had a thousand patients similarly attacked, not one in one hundred out of the thousand would be carried off, assuming, of course, the medical treatment recommended by me be implicitly observed, and that I have the patient under my care in the early stage of the attack,' he declared.

This was exciting news, and the Board wrote at once to ask Mr Blandford to appear before them the very next day. Sadly, Mr Blandford was obliged to send his regrets: a broken leg prevented him from waiting upon them. Undeterred, the Board wrote back by return asking the doctor to name a day when he expected to be able to attend. Unfortunately, however, Mr Blandford could not say when he might be well enough. The Board's next letter was to His Majesty's Navy, asking if it had ever heard of Mr Blandford. The Naval Commissioners confirmed that Mr Blandford had indeed served as an assistant surgeon in the East Indies, from 1804 to 1809, but a careful examination of his records revealed that he had never encountered a single case of cholera.

Another medical man, surgeon-apothecary Edward Bowden of Chelsea, found Sir Henry and his colleagues rather more at a loss for a reply than Mr Blandford had done. Mr Bowden had been thinking about Jenner's revolutionary practice of vaccination, not in terms of experiments but rather in terms of its normal and by then widespread use. Could there possibly be any side-effects from immunisation? he wondered. And if so, might those side-effects somehow manifest themselves as cholera? 'Is it impossible that the variolas [smallpox] poison, being restrained by vaccination from exerting what may be called its legitimate effects . . . may be driven to other structures [of the body] and spend its fury upon them?' Mr Bowden asked. The Board, with absolutely no clue as to the answer, passed swiftly on.

Meanwhile down in Sheerness on the Kent coast, nimbyism was raising its ugly head. The residents were furious at plans to offload quarantined goods in their port and store them in local ware-houses. Their MP, Thomas Law Hodges, took up the matter. What about Chertsey Hill instead? Mr Hodges suggested. He received short shrift. Ships could not get in close enough to unload at Chertsey Hill – besides which the place was extremely unhealthy, which was why the government had had the existing quarantine buildings there pulled down some years before. In any case, Sheerness would only be used as a last resort. Mr Hodges and his constituents were then treated to a lecture on their social responsi-bilities: 'If under extreme circumstances, any particular district is to oppose regulations for the general benefit of the country, it will be in vain to attempt any safe system of quarantine,' they were told.

While Mr Hodges and the inhabitants of Sheerness fretted over the prospect of potentially lethal cargoes being stockpiled in their midst, doctors, magistrates, clergymen and other local worthies in coastal towns and villages all over the United Kingdom were keeping a worried look-out for the first signs of an exotic, mystery illness. Some thirty years earlier, citizens on England's south coast had kept an equally anxious vigil for the first signs of another much-feared foreign invader called Napoleon Bonaparte.

There was a nasty scare at Port Glasgow when a twenty-five-year-old labourer, John Murray, described as previously healthy and of sober habits, died of what his doctor, John Marshall, considered a highly suspicious disease. Soon afterwards, Murray's girlfriend, Nancy Kitchen, and a friend, James McLauchlerne, 'a stout, temperate man' according to Marshall, who had sat up with the dead man during his last night, were attacked with similar symptoms of vomiting and diarrhoea. Then there was a fourth case, for which Dr Marshall said he feared that he himself had been the source: 'My own wife, who was in perfect health on the night of the 7th of July, began to complain at about 9 a.m. of the 8th. By midday, the characteristic symptoms of this appalling malady had appeared in their most frightful form. She is in person very small and delicately made, yet during the paroxysms . . . it took two strong people to keep her in bed.' But despite these sufferings so graphically described by her husband, Mrs Marshall, along with Kitchen and McLauchlerne, was happily restored to health within days. Dr Marshall, however, by now convinced that he had made the medical discovery of the decade, was off on a mission, diagnosing more and more cases of *cholera morbus* among his patients.

Seriously worried, and with the sick list in Port Glasgow growing by the hour, the Board despatched Drs Daun and Badenoch, both of whom had wide experience of cholera in India, with orders to carry out an immediate investigation. Their enquiries did not last long. The pair dismissed Dr Marshall's claims almost upon their arrival, with Dr Badenoch attributing the illness in question to the rather more mundane cause of eating too many new potatoes and fresh herrings, a common occurrence in Glasgow at that time of the year, he explained, adding: 'I have no hesitation in saying that he [Dr Marshall] came to his conclusions too rapidly and on no adequate data.'

The death in Hull the following month of forty-two-year-old

Private Martin McKeal caused another fright, and this time Dr
Daun was not so fast to rule out *cholera morbus*. After receiving a
letter from Dr Mahony, army surgeon to the Seventh Fusiliers, the
Board of Health sent Robert Daun off to Hull almost as soon as he
had returned from Port Glasgow: 'You will be good enough to
make the most explicit enquiry as to the habits of the soldier in
question, the circumstances immediately proceeding his illness, the
situation of the barracks and the possible communication with the
shipping of Hull,' Daun's instructions ran.

Private McKeal, who had been in the army for twenty years, was
considered by his superiors to be a sober, well-behaved man. On 8
August, however, he was given leave to stay out of barracks for two
nights to go to a local fair when he seems to have acted somewhat
out of character. 'By his own confession, it appears that he passed
the whole of that night in drinking and debauchery,' ran Daun's
later report. 'The succeeding night was spent in the same manner,
and so great was the quantity of ardent spirits, porter, ale, etc.,
which he drank on this night that it was remarked with astonishment by his companions in debauchery. He returned to the
barracks on Wednesday morning with his eyes bloodshot and with
bloated countenance, and in that sottish state of mind which they
who have seen much of soldiers must have often remarked to
follow a state of long-continued intoxification. In this condition, he
threw himself on the ground in the open air and fell asleep under a
hot sun.'

Despite such behaviour, which clearly upset Dr Daun, Private
McKeal still managed to find enough energy to go back to the fair
for a third night's revelling, where he spent the evening dancing and
eating large quantities of fruit, but this time drinking just a few
glasses of gin. He returned to his barracks at midnight in good spirits and quite sober, and went straight to bed. At 4 a.m., he was seized
with a violent illness and seventeen hours later he was dead.

From Dr Mahony's description, Daun considered that McKeal's
symptoms 'exhibited all the peculiar features of the malignant epidemic cholera of India', but then the doctor learnt of the soldier's

riotous last nights. This, in Daun's view, put the matter in an entirely different light. 'This case would have appeared to me as of a very suspicious character, had I not been made acquainted with the kind of life the deceased had led for the three days immediately preceeding the attack,' he explained. As it was, he saw no cause for alarm. No other cases had occurred in either the garrison or the town; the crews aboard the ships in the quarantine station remained remarkably healthy, and the huge public anxiety that the death had caused subsided as the people of Hull heard the welcome news that Private McKeal had – his doctors were now quite certain – died from drink.

On into the autumn, as the British continued to agonise over suspicious ailments in their midst, the *cholera morbus* maintained its progress westwards across Continental Europe. On 9 September, the Foreign Office received a despatch from George Chad, His Majesty's *chargé d'affaires* in Berlin, announcing that a committee of doctors had just voted by a majority of four to three that a boatman who died suddenly in his barge on the river in the busiest part of the city had been the victim of Asiatic cholera. Mr Chad then went on to relate a tragi-comic tale:

> The boatman was to be buried down the river near Spandau. Three men, pointed out by the police as persons capable of understanding what is considered a very perilous task, were employed to place the corpse in a little bark at midnight, to convey it to the appointed spot and bury it. Their courage, however, required to be so continually supported by brandy that they became unfit for their task, and in endeavouring to go through with it, they upset the boat and were all drowned.

The *chargé* then scribbled a hasty postscript to say that five new cases of cholera and one death had occurred since he wrote his letter the previous night. A week later, the Berlin death toll was fifty-eight, and a leading doctor was predicting 200 to 250 deaths a day in that city before the next week was out. In a scenario reminiscent of

St Petersburg, Chad noted that the Prussian poor were convinced that there was no such disease as cholera, but that the government had ordered the doctors to poison them because they were becoming too numerous and unruly. They also thought that this particular method of culling had been chosen because the British had previously used it with so much success in India. The Prussian king's decision to pay a special daily fee to any doctor who devoted himself to treating cholera patients did nothing to quell the rumours: the medical men were receiving a bribe for every death they caused, the tale ran.

One of the Berlin victims was a physician called Calaw whose colourful attempts to prove that the disease was not contagious ended in disaster. Mr Chad was intriguingly coy about the exact nature of Dr Calaw's scientific endeavours when he told Lord Palmerston what had happened: 'In order to establish his opinion, he had made some very disgusting experiments upon his own person, caught the malady and died of it yesterday after a few hours' illness.'

By mid-September, Francis Forbes, British Plenipotentiary in Vienna, was reporting over 300 cases of cholera in that city, with 130 deaths. A week later another 575 cases had been diagnosed, and another 220 people had died. 'I imagine that these reports can only include those who were carried to the hospitals, as many more are said to have died in their own houses,' Forbes told London.

Forbes's fellow diplomat, Henry Canning, Consul-General in Hamburg, had watched the events unfold in Berlin and Vienna with growing alarm. Britain's huge trade with the Baltic ports meant that should cholera ever appear in Canning's city, its passage across the North Sea was virtually assured. On 7 October, Canning wrote an official report informing London that Hamburg and its surrounding districts remained free of disease, but at the same time he sent a second letter marked 'Private' to Sir George Shee, Under-Secretary of State at the Foreign Office, which told a different story.

> In addition to what I have said in my public despatch [he wrote],
> I think it right to communicate to you privately . . . that a death
> occurred here yesterday which might have been suspicious if the
> physicians had not since decided that it was not a case of cholera.
> It was of a person addicted to drink, in a house inhabited by the
> lowest class of people . . . Another person under similar circum-
> stances is ill in the same house but is not yet dead. The chief
> magistrate of police from whom I obtained this information
> today qualified it strongly with the assurance that it was not
> indicative of cholera . . . Nevertheless, I feel it my decided duty to
> acquaint you with what I have heard.

The careful, stock-in-trade diplomatic language masked the anxiety
that had prompted the consul to take such a step.

At 1.30 the next afternoon, Canning wrote another, rather more
hasty, letter to Palmerston, informing him that the second person
taken ill in the house had now died, and that the news had 'created
here a great deal of suspicion'. Doctors were to examine the bodies
later that day, he said, 'but in the interval I feel it my duty to lose
no time in communicating to your Lordship what I have learnt,
and I send this by express to Cuxhaven in the hope of its being in
time to overtake the packet which is appointed to sail from thence
tomorrow morning.'

At nine o'clock that night Canning sent his second express of the
day to London. Even as he wrote, the physicians in Hamburg were
huddled together behind closed doors, trying to decide what to do. He
had managed to speak to two of them earlier that evening, and they
both told him they firmly believed that the suspicious cases – of which
there were now five, four of them already fatal – were definitely
cholera. Canning had therefore decided to issue only partial Bills of
Health to ships and passengers leaving Hamburg for British ports, but
the masters of two vessels bound for Hull refused to accept such
equivocal documents and had set off without any papers. 'I have written to the master of transit to caution him against allowing any person
to leave these vessels,' Canning warned London.

At 11.30 p.m., the lights were still burning at the British consulate in Hamburg as a frantic Canning despatched his third express in less than twenty-four hours. The doctors had just emerged to announce that the deaths bore all the worst signs of the *cholera morbus*, and although they decided to wait for further cases before making it official that the disease had reached their city, no one was any longer in the slightest doubt about the matter. To the British, watching helplessly from across the North Sea, there seemed now no chance of escape.

On 22 October 1831, the *Lancet* made a dramatic announcement: 'The cholera, that fierce and unsparing scourge of the living generation, which seems destined to sweep from the face of the earth those victims which the ruthless wars of wicked legislators have spared – the cholera . . . is now but six-and-thirty hours passage from our own shores.' Once again, however, the disease was one step ahead. As the Fleet Street presses of Messrs Mills, Jowett and Mills were busy thumping out the latest edition of the famous medical journal, the 'fierce and unsparing scourge' had already taken up residence on British soil.

CHAPTER 2

A Desperate Search

Although the next north-easterly should bear us the cholera on its wings, printers and publishers have reason to rejoice at the very rumours of its advent. Paternoster Row is in an uproar. Waggon-loads of manuscripts pour in at one end and carts full of tracts, treatises and folios issue from the other.

Lancet, 1831

The news that Tsar Nicholas's Government was to offer the world's medical elite the chance to win a prize of 25,000 roubles or £1,100 (now over £50,000) for the best essay on the *cholera morbus* caused quite a stir. Desperation was clearly running high in the Empire, although the omission of French doctors from the list of those eligible to compete showed that, even with a deadly invader at their door, there were limits to those with whom the Russians were prepared to do business.

The award was advertised in the British press and provoked an excited discussion at the next meeting of London's Westminster Medical Society, where the illustrious members expressed themselves astounded and also somewhat confused. The Russians, clearly wanting their money's worth, were specifying that the treatise had to address not only the nature of the disease, but also its causes, its method of propagation, experiments showing whether or not it was contagious, instruction on how to ward off that contagion should it prove to exist – and, of course, a definitive guide to treatment.

The Westminster Medical, as it was known, was taken aback not only at the Russians' largesse but also at what it saw as their astonishing ignorance. Countless expert studies had been published over the years on every possible aspect of the *cholera morbus*, including weighty tomes from the authorities in Bengal, Bombay and Madras. The Madras volume ran to over 700 pages and, the society's members agreed, contained some excellent information, particularly about treatment. How could the Russians possibly not know about the Indian material? Dr James Johnson told the meeting that he had already shown the Tsar's English medical adviser a list of all the relevant literature and the man confessed that he had not heard of one-quarter of it. Johnson's colleagues were suitably shocked at this revelation, one of them suggesting that the likely reason the adviser had found himself so lamentably out of touch with developments at the cutting edge of medical science was that he had spent the previous fourteen months in Yorkshire.

Yet for all their metropolitan sophistication and despite the hundreds of thousands of words that had poured out of India on the subject of the cholera, the members of the Westminster Medical were as much at a loss for definite answers about this terrifying new sickness as were the Tsar's adviser, the Russian Medical Faculty and leading physicians the world over. Where, exactly, had it come from? And after so many years confined to Asia, why had it chosen this moment to attack Europe? How was it spreading? How precisely did it act upon the body? Until some of these questions had been answered, science could not begin to tackle those that mattered most: how to cure it or, at least, how to prevent it spreading.

No one was even sure that they were dealing with one disease. Was the pestilence now attacking Russia the same one that had devastated India, as Lord Heytesbury believed? When the India veteran Dr Russell first set eyes on the St Petersburg victims, he was convinced that the two diseases were identical; but the editor of the *Lancet* was irritated that the Russians had made this assumption when they announced their prize. The advertisement was headed 'Cholera Morbus', but this term was generic, while the disease raging in Russia was specific. The *Lancet* argued: 'The first point on which information is required [by the Russia government] is "the nature of the disease" . . . The second point is "the cause which gives rise to it". To what? Certainly not the cholera of any country, but the cholera which prevails in Russia.'

With no knowledge of the living organisms responsible for so much disease and no recourse to the modern pathology laboratory or to investigations such as scans and X-rays, the business of identifying different diseases in the first half of the nineteenth century was distinctly hit-and-miss, based partly on those clinical signs that the doctor was able to see or feel for himself and partly on the patient's subjective description of the symptoms. Throughout history, bubonic plague's hideous black swellings had been only too distinctive, but for hundreds of years doctors had confused typhus and typhoid – hence their similar names – although their causes, how they are transmitted and even some of their symptoms are very different.

And while cholera, or 'the Blue Death' as it was sometimes called, was horribly unmistakable, few European doctors had ever encountered it. They had, however, come across any number of cases of stomach upsets – known confusingly in Britain as English or common cholera. The scope for mistaking a bad case of the 'English' for the real thing was considerable when the doctor didn't know what on earth he was looking for, as the enthusiastic Dr Marshall in Port Glasgow found out to his cost.

To help clear up this confusion over symptoms, Drs Russell and Barry wrote a detailed description of *cholera morbus* for the Board of Health, based partly on the pair's observations in St Petersburg. Their report, published in the *London Gazette* for all to see, made fearsome reading:

> Giddiness; sick stomach; nervous agitation; intermittent, slow or small pulse; cramps, beginning at the tops of the fingers and toes and rapidly approaching the trunk, give the first warning.

Vomiting or purging, or both these evacuations, of a liquid like rice-water or whey, or barley water, come on; the features become sharp and contracted; the eye sinks; the look is expressive of terror and wildness, as if it were a consciousness on the part of the sufferer that the hand of death is upon him; the lips, face, hands and feet, and soon after, the thighs, arms and whole surface assume a leaden, blue, purple, black or deep brown tint . . .

The fingers and toes are reduced at least a third in thickness; the skin and soft parts covering them are wrinkled, shrivelled and folded; the nails put on a bluish pearly white; the large superficial veins are marked by flat lines of a deeper black; the pulse becomes either small as a thread and scarcely vibrating, or else totally extinct.

The skin is deadly cold and often damp, the tongue always moist, often white and loaded, but flabby and chilled like a piece of dead flesh. The voice is nearly gone . . . The patient speaks in a plaintive whisper, he tosses incessantly from side to side and complains of intolerable weight and anguish around his heart. He struggles for breath, asks only for water and often lays his hand on his stomach and chest to point out the seat of his agony. Sometimes there are rigid spasms of the legs, thighs and loins . . .

Friction removes the blue colour for a time from the part rubbed; but in other parts, particularly the face, the livor becomes every moment more intense and more general. The lips and cheeks sometimes puff out and flap in expiration, with a white froth between them . . . If blood be obtained in this state, it is black, flows by drops, is thick and feels to the finger colder than natural.

Towards the close of this scene, the respiration becomes very slow, there is a quivering among the tendons of the wrist . . . The patient is at first unable to swallow, then becomes insensible; there never is, however, any rattle in the throat and he dies quietly after a long convulsive sob or two.

Not surprising, then, that in parts of South Asia such an end was known as 'mort de chien'; in other words, the victim died like a dog. Stories about what cholera could do were partly why people in nineteenth-century Britain – who lived with the constant threat of a whole host of diseases such as typhoid, typhus, smallpox, influenza and scarlet fever – regarded cholera with a fear and loathing all of its own. Another reason was that *cholera morbus* was new, foreign and quite different from anything ever seen in the country before. One doctor summed it up:

> Our other plagues were home-bred and part of ourselves, as it were; we had a habit of looking at them with fatal indifference ... But the cholera was something outlandish, unknown, monstrous; its tremendous ravages, so long foreseen and feared, so little to be explained, its insidious march over whole continents, its apparent defiance of all the known and conventional precautions against the spread of epidemic disease, invested it with a mystery and a terror which thoroughly took hold of the public mind, and seemed to recall the memory of the great epidemics of the Middle Ages.

And, of course, there was the speed with which it could kill.

Russell and Barry had produced a useful, if horrible, guide to diagnosis for the ignorant doctor and layman alike, but on the question of where the cholera 'poison' had originated or how it selected its victims they were unable to be so specific. Again, in working out the mechanics of how a disease spread, doctors in the early nineteenth century had to rely on their own observation and on anecdote, lacking anything that was recognisable as modern scientific method. They could only look at the circumstances under which individuals appeared to catch a disease and then speculate. Some conditions, such as gonorrhoea and syphilis, had already given up their unsavoury secrets, but nothing about the way cholera behaved made any sense. In its journey from its origins in India, it had tended to follow man's well-established routes by land and sea. And yet it would sometimes stop dead in its tracks and disappear without warning, only to return just as abruptly months later or to strike somewhere else, many miles away.

The Bombay treatise, of which the Russians appeared so ignorant, described cholera's strange machinations in India:

> The disease would sometimes take a complete circle round a village and, leaving it untouched, pass on as it were, wholly to depart from the district. Then after a lapse of weeks, or even months, it would suddenly return, and scarcely reappearing in the parts which had already undergone its ravages, would nearly depopulate the spot that had so lately congratulated itself on its escape. Sometimes, after running a long course on one side of the Ganges, it would, as if arrested by some unknown agent, stop at once, and taking a rapid sweep across the river, lay all waste on the opposite bank.

Perhaps, then, the cholera 'poison', whatever it was, might be airborne or at least have its origins in some unusual disturbance in the atmosphere. Again, the Bombay experience called this into question: 'The disease often travelled directly against the monsoon winds which blow for months in one uniform direction, proving almost to a demonstration that the cause was some emanation from the earth, rather than a peculiar state of the air.'

In the first half of the nineteenth century, there were two main schools of thought about how disease spread – contagionism and anti-contagionism or miasmatism. The contagionists believed that cholera and other epidemic diseases such as typhoid, typhus and influenza were spread through direct contact – that is, passed directly from person to person or through some medium such as clothing or bed linen – which was of course true for some diseases such as influenza, tuberculosis and smallpox.

The anti-contagionist credo had existed since the Middle Ages. This held that most disease stemmed from filth: in particular, from the stench, or 'miasma', given off by excrement and rotting flesh and vegetable matter (and there was plenty of all of this around in the nineteenth century), which contained poisons that made people ill. And some doctors thought that it was this very miasma, this bad gas, which was responsible for all the 'fevers'– typhoid, typhus, yellow fever and cholera – and that the extent to which a particular disease prevailed depended on some additional factor, such as the weather.

For centuries people had therefore sought protection by warding off bad smells – hence the reference to the 'pocket full o'posies' in the nursery rhyme about the plague. In the sixteenth century, Henry VIII had advised Cardinal Wolsey to 'fly to clene air incontinently' if he wanted to avoid the sweating sickness. The miasma belief had survived for so long largely because of the compelling circumstantial evidence: disease was clearly far more rampant in the stinking hovels of the poor than in the palaces of the rich. There was obviously some sort of link between dirt and disease, although no one understood what it was.

The theory about the disinfectant properties of chlorine gas, for example, which the Board of Health was finally to reject, was based largely upon its powers as an air-freshner. And when in early 1832, cholera was said to have broken out in London, it was miasmatism that prompted the Devon surgeon Thomas Calley to announce excitedly that he had found 'a ready and easy means of preventing the dreadful destruction which inevitably must follow the spreading of that disease in so populous a place'. Calley's plan was to fire off bags of gunpowder from large cannons at strategic sites around the capital such as Greenwich, the Tower of London and the Temple Gardens. The result would be the complete purification of the city's atmosphere, Calley believed: 'Every man knows who has been in the habit of shooting that not only his clothes are impregnated with the gas, but it travels through every channel of his body, and my opinion is that it offers as good a preventative against contagion as anything yet known – an infant may inhale it.'

Florence Nightingale, who was to nurse hundreds of cholera cases among the troops in the Crimea in the mid-1850s, was a convinced miasmatist all her life and a firm believer in the powers of fresh air. 'The very first cannon of nursing, the first and last thing upon which a nurse's attention must be fixed, the first essential to the patient, without which all the rest you can do for him is as nothing, with which I had almost said you may leave all the rest alone, is this: To keep the air he breathes as pure as the external air without chilling him,' she insisted. And of 'the fatal effects of the effluvia from excreta,' Miss Nightingale added, 'it would seem unnecessary to speak.'

Cholera, however, was so confusing that not everyone was firmly in either the contagionist or miasmatist camp about this disease. Its long trek across Asia and into Europe, following the main trade routes, seemed to point clearly to contagion, but then what of the Bombay experience, where it appeared able to jump where it would, without any need for human intervention? And what of the countless cases where people caring for the sick and dying – breathing their air, washing their bodies, cleaning up their vomit – had emerged unscathed?

Dr Walker, whom Ambassador Heytesbury had sent to Moscow with instructions to pronounce on the contagion question, had come across any number of such seemingly miraculous examples, but decided to hedge his bets when he reported back to London. 'I believe it is capable of being conveyed from one place to another by men,' he wrote, 'although it cannot be considered completely proven; while, although it is not evidence sufficient to prove its communication by clothes or goods, still we cannot say that it is impossible.' In other words, Walker, despite his £5-a-day-plus-expenses fact-finding mission, remained as confused as everyone else, and his less than enlightening conclusions led Sir Charles Greville, secretary to the Privy Council, to pronounce him 'a very useless and inefficient agent'. Walker proved no more effective when he tried to interest the Russians in a novel plan of Sir William Pym's, which the Superintendent General of Quarantine believed might settle the contagion issue once and for all. Criminals under sentence of death could be allowed to escape execution if they

agreed to wear the soiled clothes and sleep in the foul bedding
of people who had died from cholera, Sir William suggested. This
idea proved a touch too distasteful even for robust nineteenth-
century nerves, however and, besides, as Walker explained, capital
punishment was then virtually non-existent in Russia.

In the meantime, the baffled medical profession devised countless convoluted theories, weaving together different aspects of
contagionism and anti-contagionism, trying to come up with an
answer that would fit all of the contradictory facts. Some doctors
proposed that the disease was not normally contagious but that it
could become so in circumstances such as poor hygiene or overcrowding, while others thought a chemical or electrical disturbance
in the atmosphere might be involved, coming either from the air or
from deep in the earth. Or perhaps a victim's physical state or
lifestyle were partly to blame – an excess of carbon in the body, for
example, or that favourite scapegoat, over-indulgence in alcohol,
particularly, of course, among the feckless lower classes.

James Johnson, who had accused *The Times* of sensationalism
and who, like Dr Russell, had come across cholera in India many
years earlier, agreed with the Bombay report that the disease had
its main origins under the ground, and he thought that it then
emerged to pollute the atmosphere: 'I am perfectly convinced that,
although . . . under certain unfavourable circumstances, it [cholera]
may take on a contagious or infectious character . . . the primary
cause springs from the bowels of the earth, and thus contaminates
the air we breathe . . . The mysterious, I had almost said capricious,
courses which cholera has hitherto pursued, destroy entirely the
idea of contagion as its general cause,' Johnson insisted. Russell
himself had been a non-contagionist during his India days, but his
experiences in St Petersburg changed his mind. Events in the
Russian capital, he said, 'have a good deal shaken my belief as to
the disease not being communicable by persons or effects. It seems
tolerably well ascertained that cholera has not broken out spontaneously in any place without communication by persons or effects
coming from infected places.'

The maddeningly elusive answer to this question of contagion did not just preoccupy the medical profession: the worlds of politics and commerce also had a huge interest in the matter but for rather different reasons. Quarantine restricts the free movement of goods, disrupts trade, puts companies out of business and people out of work, and generally damages a country's economy. If cholera were not capable of being passed on by individuals or, more importantly, carried in cargo, then such a ruinous measure as quarantine was pointless. In September 1831, a furious Lord Palmerston had ordered Francis Forbes, the Foreign Office's man in Vienna, to remonstrate with the Austrian Chancellor Prince Metternich over the quarantines imposed on ships arriving at some of the Adriatic ports. Forbes was to inform His Highness that not one single case of *cholera morbus* had appeared in any part of the United Kingdom and to call His Highness's attention to the 'extraordinary and needless restrictions' put upon on British vessels, not to mention the scandalous quarantine fees. Metternich took the point, and a delighted Mr Forbes was soon reporting back to London that an exception was henceforth to be made for ships from British ports. Sadly though, in boasting about the excellent state of his country's health, Palmerston had spoken too soon.

Britain had itself been enforcing a strict quarantine on all ships from infected foreign ports since June 1831. On 20 October, however, with cholera now officially just over the water, the Privy Council published a long list of Sir Henry Halford's new measures aimed largely at trying to contain the disease, should it succeed in landing. The regulations were prefaced by some solemn remarks that can have done little to lift the spirits of a frightened nation. 'The measures of external precaution for preventing the introduction of the cholera morbus by a rigorous quarantine have hitherto been found effectual,' their Lordships allowed. 'But as the disease approaches the neighbouring shores, not only is the necessity of increased vigilance more apparent, but it is also consistent with common prudence that the country should be prepared to meet the possible contingency of so dreadful a calamity.' Clearly, optimism was in short supply at the Privy Council.

Every town and village, starting with those on the coast, was told
to set up its own local board of health, consisting of magistrates,
clergy, doctors and other prominent local citizens. In the coastal
areas, one of the boards' tasks would be to make sure that the residents understood just what a terrible risk they ran if they continued
to engage in the popular local pastime of smuggling. Another of the
boards' duties was to inform London the moment they uncovered a
case of the disease, and here Barry and Russell's terrifying guide to
symptoms would prove useful. The boards were also to set aside
buildings to which the sick could be quickly removed, and if any
refused to go – for, unlike the tsarist authorities, the British government had no powers to force its people into hospital – then the
word 'Sick' was to be prominently displayed outside their homes.
And no chances were to be taken with the victims' houses and
possessions:

Decayed articles, such as rags, cordage, papers, old clothes,
hangings should be burnt. Filth of every description removed;
clothing and furniture should be submitted to copious effusions
of water, and boiled in a strong ley [a caustic solution]; drains
and privies thoroughly cleansed by streams of water and chloride
of lime; . . . the walls of the house, from the cellar to the garret,
should be hot lime-washed; all loose and decayed pieces of plas-
tering should be removed.

Then, with more than a nod in the direction of miasmatism, Sir
Henry's Board went on: 'It is impossible to impress too strongly
the necessity of extreme cleanliness and free ventilation. They are
points of the very greatest importance, whether in the houses of
the sick, or generally as a measure of precaution.' But with the
possibility of contagion still also firmly in mind, Sir Henry
and his colleagues announced that the dead were to be banned
from the churchyards and buried in separate grounds close to the
cholera hospitals, 'so as to confine as much as possible every
source of infection to one spot'. For the same reason, as few people

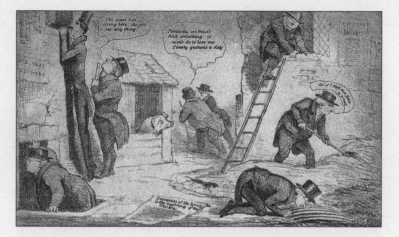

A local board of health trying to track down cases of cholera,
as seen by a cartoonist in 1832

as possible were to be involved in nursing patients and transporting them to hospital, and those who did do this work would
have to move away from their homes and families and live apart
from the rest of the community. All contact with an infected
town must be broken off at once, and the local magistrates would
have to draw up regulations under which food could be brought
in. However, Sir Henry warned, if so fatal a disease did ever
show itself in Britain, then even tougher measures might be
needed; for example, troops or police could be drafted in to
enforce the cordons, although the Board said they felt sure that if
this were to happen, the people would willingly accept it for the
safety of the State.

The *Lancet*, no fan of the Board of Health, whose members it
had once described as 'an assemblage of wiseacres [dunces], not
less ridiculous for their want of knowledge upon the subject they
are called upon to investigate', was excoriating about the last plan,
which appears to have been leaked to the press before its official
publication:

We perceive by a paragraph in the newspapers – which has probably been put forth by some exceedingly active and diligent
member of the Board of Health, who is anxious to prove to the
public that he and his co-adjudicators are doing something for
the £500 a year which Sir Henry Halford has procured for
them – that the Board intends to recommend that such places as
may be attacked in this country should be isolated from the rest
of the community. Sagacious legislators, who cannot prevent the
cholera from traversing the ocean, yet can keep it from pene-
trating a hedge or crossing a field!

The point was unanswerable; it was simply that no one else, the
razor-penned *Lancet* writer included, could think of a better idea.

And there was just as much disagreement over the question of
treatment. Again, there was no shortage of well-argued theories
and case histories: the number of clinical papers on the subject
ran into thousands, while the lists of remedies and regimens
could be measured by the yard. The only problem was that none
of it seemed to work. In the first half of the nineteenth century,
medical treatment had advanced little since the Middle Ages.
Much of it was not only useless but barbarous, and sometimes
even fatal. The list of remedies for cholera patients ranged from
bleeding to hot poultices applied to the abdomen and boiling
water to the feet; enemas of every description, normally with the
instruction that they were to be 'thrown well up'; and draughts
of medicine containing ingredients such as ammonia, oils,
pepper, spices, *nux vomica*, camphor, turpentine, sulphuric acid,
creosote, bismuth (a metal whose salts were also used to treat
syphilis), and a herb, catechu. The doctors' particular favourites
were a deadly compound called calomel, which could destroy
patients' gums and intestines before finally killing them from
mercury poisoning; and laudanum, a blend of opium and brandy
that cured nothing but, unlike the rest of the potions, at least
made the symptoms easier to bear. It was not that the doctors
were especially careless or irresponsible, but rather that they

had nothing else to offer, and desperate cases led to desperate measures.

The inefficacy, or worse, of these remedies did not curb the medical profession's enthusiasm for them in the slightest. In the 1880s, looking back over a long and illustrious medical career, Sir James Paget was to describe how doctors dealt with cholera in 1831: 'Observations on the effects of treatment were vaguely made, not exactly recorded, not tabulated and the principles were deemed sure, whatever consequences might ensue from observations of them.' As Paget pointed out, with little attempt at measuring the results of the doctors' efforts, who could be certain what use they were? If a patient died, the doctor could claim this had been a hopeless case from the start, but if he or she recovered, was this thanks to medical care or despite it?

As long ago as ten years before this outbreak, the naval surgeon Sir Gilbert Blane, who served in the American War of Independence and helped to introduce lime juice into the sailors' diet to prevent scurvy, had urged doctors to try to assess just what it was they were achieving for their patients and then to base their future treatments on that evidence. 'Unless we can calculate with some degree of precision the extent of the powers of nature, we shall find it impossible to assign what is due to them and what to the agency of medicine,' he wrote. 'For without such discrimination, we may not be able to satisfy ourselves whether recoveries have been effected by virtue of medicine or in spite of it . . . and we run the risk of congratulating ourselves on a great cure where there may have only been a happy escape.'

For three-year-old Londoner William Somerville, there was to be no happy escape. The child was a tragic example of what could, and sometimes did, go wrong in medicine. William had what was described as a fever – probably in this case some mild infection – and his washerwoman mother asked the advice of one of her customers, 'a young medical gentleman', who gave her twelve white powders all to be taken within twenty-four hours. They contained huge doses of mercury. No sooner had the boy taken them than his face swelled up, his gums went black and his teeth began falling out. Two days later a small black spot appeared on his chin and started to spread over his entire face. Five days after William swallowed the first powder, all of his teeth were gone, his face was black, his right eye closed and 'the little fellow [was] moaning constantly', wrote one of the doctors at Westminster Hospital where the child was taken. William died just a week after receiving his 'treatment' for an illness that might well have cleared up by itself.

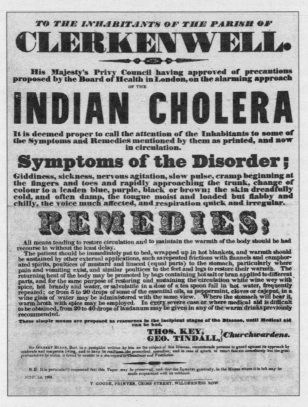

A London Parish poster warning of cholera symptoms and giving advice on remedies, 1831

While the Board of Health waited for reports from people like Drs Russell, Barry and Walker on the latest cholera therapies in Europe, it published some advice on the subject from India. This said that the physician's first aims should be to 'rally the animal powers' by means of heat and internal and external stimulation; and to stop the vomiting, diarrhoea and muscle spasms with opium and other sedatives. The next step was to ease the laboured breathing and 'restore the passage of bile' – the doctors were much struck by the fact that the bile, or yellowy secretions from the liver, usually seen in the vomit and excreta of patients with ordinary stomach disorders, including the so-called 'English cholera', was absent in *cholera morbus*, and they believed this to be significant.

In India the sick were usually first given opium, followed as soon as the vomiting had stopped by combinations of different types of strong laxatives, of which calomel was usually the main ingredient. The opium might be given in the form of sixty to eighty drops of laudanum – then readily available in Britain, used for practically every ailment known to man and to which many people were addicted – or an equivalent amount of solid opium. Calomel was prescribed in doses of ten, fifteen or twenty grains or more, to be repeated once every two, three or four hours. The other favourite purgatives included jalapium, scammonium, colocynth and croton oil – all powerful plant extracts found in Asia, the Middle East and Central America; as well as rhubarb, senna, metallic salts, magnesia and, particularly, castor oil.

At the same time, the patient was given medicine intended to warm the body and boost the circulation, such as brandy and other spirits, ether, ammonia and oil of peppermint. Assafoetida, a plant from Iran believed to stop involuntary muscular spasms, was often prescribed for the cramps, either alone or combined with opium, while turpentine was given as a liquid enema, known as a clyster, squirted into the rectum. Cajeput oil was also reportedly used to good effect. Cajeput is a green, camphor-like substance from the leaves of a tree native to India and was widely prescribed for chronic and painful diseases.

Much of the so-called external stimulation was based on the principle of counter-irritation; in other words, causing a superficial irritation to try to relieve a deeper irritation, either generally in the body or in a particular organ. This could be done with dry heat, such as bottles of hot water or sand applied to the skin; moist heat in the form of hot-water baths or vapour baths, blistering plasters or poultices to various parts of the body; or mechanically, through brisk rubbing, usually with linaments such as camphor or turpentine.

Blistering plasters were prepared by heating a known irritant such as mustard to scalding point, spreading it on to linen or silk, and then slapping it on to the body so that the heat and irritant together would burn the skin. In India, cantharides plasters were often applied to the pit of the stomach, where the seat of the problem was believed to lie. Cantharides, or Spanish flies, are greeny-gold insects, prepared for medicinal use by being gassed with sulphur fumes and then dried in a stove, thus rendering them 'one of the best and most powerful of all medical remedies', according to the 1807 *Edinburgh Medical and Physical Dictionary*. The active ingredient, cantharidin, is indeed powerful: as well as acting as a skin irritant, when taken internally it is both a diuretic and an aphrodisiac – and also, in higher doses, a deadly poison.

If the patient was in a virtual state of collapse, however, stronger measures were called for, and so boiling water was used instead. At first it might appear harsh to pour boiling water on to a patient's abdomen, as the London surgeon Mr Boye acknowledged during an earnest discussion at the Westminster Medical Society, but in order to be beneficial the treatment had to be both prompt and vigorous.

In London that autumn, Dr James Johnson demonstrated a new piece of equipment designed to stimulate circulation in cholera sufferers. It consisted of an arched basketwork frame with small apertures in the sides and blankets draped over the top, which was placed over the patient. One end of the frame was closed off by a board with a hole in it, just big enough to admit a tube. The other end of the tube was connected to a spirit lamp, so that the patients in their wicker boxes were encased in steady clouds of scalding steam. At the same time, attendants could put their gloved hands through the holes to apply the necessary friction. While this procedure was underway, the patients were also to be given calomel as a laxative and mustard or sulphate of zinc to make them vomit.

However, the treatment most highly regarded by the doctors in India was that to which virtually the entire medical profession seemed completely wedded – namely, bleeding. A thickening and blackening of the blood, which was often described as tar-like, was another of cholera's hideous trademarks, and while it made bleeding difficult and sometimes impossible, the doctors thought that by trying to drain off this treacley substance that was clogging up the veins they might restore the body's normal free-flowing circulation. 'This practice [bleeding] seemed to apply itself to the root of the disease by relieving the congestion of the venous system, which was invariably found loaded on examination after death,' the Board of Health explained, adding that the recommended amount of blood to be drawn was eighteen, twenty-four or thirty ounces.

Thus people already dying an agonising death also ran the risk of being boiled, steamed and scalded; of having the linings of their mouths, stomachs and intestines seared with acid and their systems poisoned with deadly metallic salts, while draughts of blood were drained from their arms, powerful emetics poured down their throats and substances like turpentine squirted into their rectums.

What the medical men lacked in skill and knowledge, many of them more than made up for in professional pride, and huge rows erupted over the question of treatment. An ill-tempered spat among a group of international experts in Warsaw got completely out of hand when Drs Searle and Mikulniski challenged each other to a duel by sword in order to settle the matter. One shocked onlooker lost patience with his learned colleagues: 'When such a devastating demon as this disease is making such fearful strides, it is lamentable to see men quarrelling about bismuth and calomel,' he said. 'Two of these gentlemen are thinking of fighting for the reputation of their panacea, and if they kill each other in their chivalrous tournament, they will probably not be missed in Warsaw.'

Had Searle and Mikulniski and their colleagues the world over taken an honest look at the results of their efforts, however, they would have been forced to agree with Mr Wakem of St George's Hospital, London, when he said: 'In the treatment of cholera, I have never found any medicine that I could positively say has been of any use.'

CHAPTER 3

It's Here

The conduct of the people of Sunderland was more suitable to the barbarism of the interior of Africa than to a town in a civilized country.

Charles Greville, diarist and clerk to the Privy Council, November 1831

Dr Clanny stared down at the gaunt figure before him on the heap of straw, his professional calm masking his fears. Sunderland's most eminent medical man, physician to the King's younger brother and senior consultant at the local infirmary, had been called in to give a second opinion on this forty-year-old pauper woman, and he now found himself in the most delicate as well as frightening situation.

The woman's own doctor had diagnosed typhus, but Clanny's first glance told him that this was no case of the so-called 'gaol fever', common in these filthy lanes. But the doctor noted the patient's constant vomiting and diarrhoea that had lasted for eight hours; the wracking cramps; the pinched, icy face; blue distorted fingers and toes; and the 'corrugated' skin of her hands – as though she had been washing linen. The signs all told a different story. And although Clanny, in over forty years of medicine, had never yet come across a case of the notorious *cholera morbus*, the scene before him was, he felt sure, indisputable proof of what the town, and the whole country with it, so dreaded and feared. No case of the disease had yet been confirmed on English soil, but it now seemed beyond dispute that the cholera had arrived and that Sunderland was its first port of call.

Earlier that summer, the physician had noted in his diary some strange happenings that he thought might have prefigured this disaster. First the neighbourhood had been invaded by great swarms of young toads, the likes of which had never before been seen in the town, and no sooner had they disappeared than the area was rocked by a series of powerful thunderstorms. And over the weeks to come, as the body count rose, the pragmatic Ulsterman William Reid Clanny, inventor of a safety lamp for miners, was also to ponder over the lightning strikes that followed the toads and the thunder. His deliberations were not based purely on superstition: the ancient Greek tradition of medicine in which Clanny was steeped taught that the weather was often linked to epidemics, and he was now struggling to apply his knowledge to this new and mysterious danger.

Now, though, he faced a more immediate dilemma. He was the most senior medical man on the local board of health, set up on the orders of Sir Henry Halford in London, and it was his duty to warn the government the moment the disease struck. As cholera moved steadily westwards across Germany that summer, Sunderland had known only too well that its huge trade with the Baltic ports just over the North Sea put it right in the firing line. Now that Hamburg had fallen, disaster seemed only a matter of days, perhaps even hours, away. Some of the townspeople were already whispering that the sickness among them was something quite different, something infinitely more terrible, than the usual, familiar stomach troubles that plagued them regularly in the autumn months. So far there had been only rumours, but Sunderland was at fever pitch, its population terrified not only at the prospect of the cholera itself but also at the financial hardship – destitution for many – from the quarantine on their port that would follow the appearance of a deadly foreign disease. A doctor would need more than his fair share of courage to diagnose a case of Asiatic cholera in this town; and, having done so, he had better be right.

'I wished to avoid giving offence to any person, but at the same time I was impelled by an ardent desire to ascertain the nature of epidemic cholera in the face of every obstacle,' Clanny later explained. 'It is well known that more than half of our medical practitioners denied that any new disease had broken out in Sunderland. For a length of time our new epidemic was called simple diarrhoea, common cholera, congestive fever, typhus, etc.'

Sunderland sits on the bank of the river Wear, ten miles south of the great commercial port of Newcastle upon Tyne, the capital of north-east England, and twelve miles from the historic cathedral-city of Durham. In 1831, the town consisted largely of two long streets, the High Street and the Low. The High Street was a broad, cheerful place, lined with well-stocked shops and generally bustling with people, while the Low was narrow and winding, following the curves of the river, and packed with building yards, breweries and anchorsmiths. Small lanes ran off the High Street at right angles, and it was here that the great mass of the working classes lived, virtually all of them employed in the coal trade: as sailors; as keelmen, bringing coals down river to the ships in the port; as casters, hurling coals on to the waiting vessels, or in one of the countless jobs essential to keeping a huge tonnage of shipping on the seas. If the weather was fair, up to 200 ships might enter the harbour at one time, and their owners, anxious to turn them around fast, paid the labourers good wages. When the winter storms set in, however, the windows of the pawnshops in the lanes quickly filled up with any trinkets that would fetch a few shillings.

The western end of the High Street ran into the district called Bishopswearmouth, home to the better-off professional classes including Dr Clanny and most of his medical colleagues. In fact, as one of the doctors remarked, scarcely anyone of any status or influence in Sunderland actually lived in the town itself. By contrast, the extreme east end of Sunderland was dominated by the great barracks, base of the 82nd reserve regiment and home to

400 men, women and children, while in front of it lay the town's slum quarter: a maze of foul-smelling alleys and tenements.

Clanny's latest patient belonged to that world, and her circumstances, as well as the fact that the first doctor had misdiagnosed her illness, made the consultant especially determined to do his best for her. He ordered a strong infusion of lean mutton to be squirted into the woman's rectum and held tightly in place with a wadded 'T'-shaped bandage: 'I directed that if the bandage were not sufficient, a tapering cork, well oiled, should be placed within the sphincter ani after a fresh injection had been thrown up.' Eight hours later – to his great relief because the use of a cork to retain a liquid enema was certainly not standard medical practice – Clanny found his patient 'much relieved in every respect'.

Little Isabella Hazard was not so lucky. The twelve-year-old lived in the Low Street near Fish Quay, where her parents ran a pub popular with the shipworkers. On Sunday, 16 October 1831, after twice attending church, Isabella went to bed in perfect health, but at midnight was suddenly struck down with vomiting, torrents of watery diarrhoea and an unquenchable thirst. Her eyes were sunk in their sockets, her features unrecognisable, her legs seized with terrible spasms, her pulse scarcely perceptible and her whole body

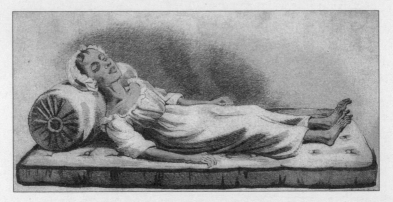

An engraving of Isabella Hazard after her death

freezing. Most alarming of all, her skin turned such a terrible dark blue that her mother asked the doctor, Mr Cook: 'What makes the child so black?' By four in the morning, Cook knew that he was out of his depth and sent for Clanny, who ordered a warm bath, brandy and hot water, mustard plasters to the legs, and an hourly dose of opium, ammonia and peppermint. On his return three hours later, the physician found no improvement in his patient's condition. He ordered the treatment to continue, however, and saw the little girl again at 11 a.m., by which time the case was clearly hopeless. Isabella died at four o'clock that afternoon.

Next to go was William Sproat, a tough sixty-year-old keelman, who had a large airy room in a house on the quayside, 'a musket-ball's throw' in local parlance, from the Hazards' pub. On Thursday night, three days after Isabella died, Dr Holmes was called out to treat him for a violent gastric illness and prescribed calomel and opium at bedtime and castor oil in the morning. A couple of days later Sproat seemed to be on the mend but then he had a violent relapse, which Dr Holmes blamed on the patient ignoring his advice about diet and having a mutton chop for dinner. By the morning of Wednesday, 26 October, Sproat was sinking fast and at noon he was dead. An hour later, his granddaughter, ten-year-old Margaret, collapsed by the corpse, and her father, William junior, 'a fine athletic young man,' according to Clanny, who had nursed his father day and night, was struck down the following day. Father and daughter were rushed to the local infirmary, where Clanny saw them both. William, he said, appeared as though he were 'in a kind of drunken debauch', thrashing wildly about and biting the bed clothes: 'A vein was freely opened and about four ounces of thick black blood was extracted, which, on being left at rest, appeared like jelly.' William died a few hours later.

The day after William and Margaret were admitted to hospital, Dr Clanny and his colleagues at the infirmary met in the boardroom to discuss the cases. They asked James Butler Kell, surgeon to the 82nd reserves and at that time the only man in town with experience of *cholera morbus*, to join the debate.

They were soon to regret their invitation. The army surgeon described what happened next:

> The highly respectable practitioners stated their belief that it was the common cholera of this country, attended with aggravated symptoms, and that many cases of the disease, equally severe and some of which proved fatal, occurred in the month of August. I then explicitly gave it as my firm conviction that the disease under which Sproat and his daughter laboured was Asiatic cholera.

Kell went on to tell the gathering that he had already reported as much to the Board of Health in London, which caused something of an uproar among the highly respectable practitioners. Kell, however, who was not a man to be thrown off course by the sensibilities of a few colleagues, then explained his reasoning to the meeting, after which he 'rested satisfied with the propriety of my proceedings'. No one else in the room was quite so happy with his conduct, however, and only Clanny agreed with his diagnosis of Asiatic cholera.

By now, on the quayside and up and down the alleys that ran between the High Street and the Low, they were dying in earnest. A fifty-six-year-old labourer named Robert Jordan who occupied a dirty basement in New Road breathed his last – like Sproat senior – on 26 October, just eleven hours after being taken ill. On Sunday, 30 October, the day before Sproat junior died, a thirty-five-year-old shoemaker called Rodenburg, who lived with his family in what his doctor described as a wretched hovel, ate a plate of pork for supper and went to bed in seemingly good health, but was then taken violently ill at about midnight. Dr Hazlewood described what happened next: 'He was attacked with . . . violent cramps of the whole body, affecting the different fingers and toes successively; his voice was quickly reduced to a whisper, nails blue, skin livid and covered with cold sweat, pulse at the wrist imperceptible . . . At 12 o'clock, when being at his own request raised up, he instantly expired.'

The post-mortem findings on Rodenburg's body make equally grim reading:

> On opening the pericardium [membrane around the heart], the interior and superior venae cavae were observed greatly distended; these vessels and all the cavities of the heart were gorged with blood of a black colour and resembling tar; the blood was adhesive to the touch; and when the ventricles were laid open, they appeared as if treacle had been poured over them ... The mucous membrane [of the stomach] was thickened and so soft as to be easily peeled off and torn with a nail. The prominent parts of the corrugations exhibited a black tinge, as if a paint brush dipped in Indian ink had been passed lightly over ... On continuing our examination downwards, the fluid [in the intestine] became much whiter, precisely resembling a strong solution of soap, and where thinner, of whey, containing numerous white flocculi. In the caput caecum coli [part of the colon] the fluid had much of resemblance to pus.

The day after Rodenburg died, another keelman, fifty-one-year-old Thomas Wilson, was struck down. One of Dr Clanny's colleagues at the infirmary, a physician called John Miller, wrote up the case notes:

> Wilson was attacked on the morning of 31 October, about 4 o'clock ... Mr Cook, surgeon, was called for at six o'clock ... At seven o'clock I was called to him; pulse at this time not distinguishable at the wrists; skin over the surface of the body cold as death; lips blue; eyes dim and sunk in the head. Did not vomit; complained of intense pain in the epigastrium and abdomen, with cramps of the extremities ... Extreme restlessness, moaning and sighing; speaks in a whisper ...
>
> The spasms ceased about nine o'clock; no vomiting or purging. There appeared a total loss of power of the nervous and circulating systems, and it appeared evident that the man must

die. I left him, and saw him again at 12 o'clock; had the appearance of a living corpse. Eyes deeply sunk in their sockets; hands and fingers remarkably shrivelled, very much reduced in size, of a light blue tinge. He gradually got worse and expired at three o'clock in the afternoon.

Wilson was followed by Eliza Turnbull, a nurse at the infirmary who died just a few hours after laying out Sproat's body. Betty Short went to her grave a week later and Robert 'Jack' Crawford, a forgotten hero of the 1797 naval Battle of Camperdown, the day after that.

The medical men did their best, putting the victims through every possible combination of torments. Betty Short, for example, whom Dr Hazlewood and a local surgeon, Mr Mordey, had discovered crouched by the fire, her knees drawn up to her chin and an overflowing bucket by her side, was subjected to what the doctors described as a very varied treatment, including brandy, laudanum, calomel, cajeput oil, rhubarb, jalap, turpentine, bleeding to eight ounces, a mustard poultice and a turpentine enema. Like Mrs Short, Robert Jordan was also dosed with brandy, laudanum, calomel and turpentine, but in addition he had to endure ammonia, sulphuric ether, scalding bricks on his feet, hands and stomach, and bladders of boiling water on his head. Rodenburg fortunately managed to escape proper medical attention for much of his illness and consequently received only brandy, laudanum and ether before he died. A visitor from London commented: 'A Chinese mandarin, who has to swallow simultaneously the separate medicines ordered by each of the scores of his physicians, was never more copiously or heterogeneously drugged as are some of these unhappy creatures.' And in nearly every case, it was all for nothing.

By now, in Dr Clanny's eyes the medical evidence in favour of Asiatic cholera was beyond dispute and the time had come for Sunderland's medical profession, and the rest of the town with it, to face up to the truth. When nurse Eliza Turnbull had virtually dropped dead in the infirmary from such a seemingly obvious source of infection as Sproat's body, panic ran through every class of Sunderland society, and it was becoming increasingly untenable for the doctors to continue diagnosing these terrible deaths as a severe form of common cholera. Clanny decided to call his colleagues together to thrash out their differences once and for all about what, exactly, it was that they were dealing with. The medical men duly met again, fresh from a post-mortem examination on the ravaged remains of the once-athletic William Sproat junior. To the consultant's great relief, this time they voted unanimously in favour of the motion he had put before them: 'We have the continental cholera among us.' It was the first such announcement on British shores.

By nightfall, Clanny's official notification, as opposed to Kell's informal report, was on its way to London and the response from the Privy Council, ready and waiting, was swift. Robert Daun, veteran of the *cholera morbus* of India, not to mention the more recent dramas of Hull and Port Glasgow, and the Board of Health's favourite safe pair of hands, arrived post-haste from the capital with his by-now familiar brief to discover just why people were sickening and dying. This time, however, the Lords of the Privy Council appeared fairly sure that they knew the answer already, for hard on Daun's heels came the redoubtable Lieutenant-Colonel Michael Creagh, later Sir Michael. Creagh's orders were clear and his resolution firm. As soon as the officer set foot in town he sought out Dr Clanny and then, after crashing in on Kell and Daun while the latter was finishing his breakfast in Kell's lodgings, announced an immediate fifteen-day quarantine on all vessels leaving the Wear for domestic ports, enforcing his proclamation by stationing a warship just offshore in case anyone was in any doubt about the matter.

Kell felt himself vindicated. His experiences of the disease in Mauritius in the 1820s had convinced him that cholera was highly contagious and could be caught from clothing and bed linen, as well as passed on by direct person-to-person contact. He had already caused a row about a river pilot called Robert Henry, who had died in September from what Kell was convinced had been

Asiatic cholera, and he had long been warning about what he saw as Sunderland's laxity over the quarantining of ships from foreign ports. He had previously called for a brig of war, or at least heavy artillery, at the entrance to the river to enforce the regulations. No one had paid much attention at the time, and even after the death of Isabella Hazard, the army surgeon had uncovered more evidence of what, to his military mind, was a severe dereliction of duty by the port authorities and a threat to 'the safety and happiness of the population of the Empire'.

At the request of one of the local surgeons, Kell had gone to see a seventeen-year-old lad called Dodds who was close to collapse. Dodds told Kell that he had been in perfect health until the previous night when he was suddenly seized with the most appalling symptoms, and it was this violent onset, so characteristic of Asiatic cholera, that worried Kell. Dodds worked in a shipwright's yard on the river bank at a place called Deptford, where several ships were anchored under quarantine, and the conscientious Kell lost no time in going to see the situation for himself. He was not reassured by what he found: 'There were three or four ships in the river with the yellow flag; the tide was out, the water shallow and from the want of a marine, police or military guard, I could not discover how the intended seclusion could be carried into effect.'

But while Kell considered Creagh's new measures to be the very least that the situation demanded, Sunderland's merchants and shipowners were outraged over what they saw as the government's ridiculous, not to say damaging, over-reaction. A week after Daun and Creagh's arrival, the local newspaper was still insisting that nothing was amiss in the town. 'That five persons expired is true, but there are doubts as to the causes of their deaths,' said the *Sunderland Herald*, 'and had it not been for the too-zealous communications of some alarmists, it is more than probable that the inhabitants of Sunderland would have been represented as having the enjoyment of more than ordinary health.'

There were no more patients than usual in the infirmary or on the local doctors' books, the paper's editor maintained. He then went on, in the best journalistic tradition, to overstate his case: 'In fact, the general appearance and gaiety of the inhabitants of these towns were never more apparent. No one hides or shuts himself up as if inhaling an atmosphere charged with deadly contagion; they assemble in groups and are as busy ... as at any former period; and the theatre continues open.' Any sickness that did exist was clearly no more than the usual maladies that affected the poor. He believed they had only themselves to blame, for he had it on good authority that that part of town where the so-called 'destructive malady' was most prevalent was 'inhabited by persons steeped in poverty through dissipation and idleness'.

Despite the strident views of the *Sunderland Herald*, clearly something of a *Daily Mail* of its time, on 8 November Colonel Creagh informed London that Daun was convinced beyond all doubt that the disease killing people in Sunderland was 'the epidemic, malignant cholera', adding that he was sorry to say that it was now spreading fast. The *Herald* was certainly right in one respect, however: the slum streets were definitely being hit hardest, a fact that Creagh, for one, found encouraging. If cholera flourished in dirt and decay, he reasoned, then controlling its spread should be an easy matter. Almost at once, the energetic colonel had the fire engines out washing down the streets, backed up by an army of men with brooms, scrubbing years of accumulated filth from the gutters and gullies. At the same time, he procured a pipe (114 gallons) of brandy and laudenam, and piles of blankets for distribution to the poor.

Both he and Daun, neither of them squeamish men, were appalled at the conditions they found tucked away behind the prosperous bustle of the High Street. 'I believe that in no other town of the Empire is there to be found a pauper population so dense as there is in some parts of Sunderland,' Daun wrote to his friend Sir Edward Seymour. 'In the lanes and narrow alleys, every room, from the cellar to the garret, contains a family averaging from four to five persons in the most abject state of poverty.' He was particularly moved by Rodenburg's pitiful home, which he

visited after the shoemaker's death: 'The room of Rodenburg measured eight feet by ten and had served the poor man as a kitchen,
boot shop and bedroom for himself, his wife and four children.'

Despite their determination, the two emissaries from London
soon found that organising a clean-up and supplying the poor with
a few creature comforts were the easier parts of their task. Blankets
and clean streets posed no threat to anyone. Obtaining accurate
medical reports and opening a designated cholera hospital, as the
Privy Council had instructed, were different matters, however, and
here the pair met with a wall of obstruction. Daun designed a form
for recording all cases of *cholera morbus*, common cholera and
simple diarrhoea. The doctors were asked to list each patient's age,
sex, symptoms, circumstances, occupation, alcohol consumption,
and whether he or she was currently sick, recovering, cured or
dead. Daun announced he would send an orderly to every doctor's
home each morning between 10 and 11 a.m. to collect the newly
completed forms for the previous day and would then use this
information to compile his own daily report for the government.

It seemed a good plan. The drawback was that the only man in
town prepared to fill in his forms with any attempt at accuracy was
Dr Clanny. And while Daun, like Creagh, was convinced that
vested commercial interests lay behind this lack of co-operation, a
few days' acquaintance with his Sunderland colleagues had him
wondering whether some of them were intellectually or medically
capable of complying with his request. He was particularly with-
ering about the parish surgeon Mr Embleton, who, to Daun's
disgust, turned out not to be a surgeon at all but a mere apothecary. 'He is evidently that sort of half-educated practitioner with
whom I would find it very unpleasant, as well as difficult, to act,'
Daun complained.

By 15 November, a full month after Isabella Hazard had died,
Daun and Creagh finally had a cholera hospital open for business,
thanks largely to the efforts of the Reverend Robert Grey, Rector of
Sunderland, who, Daun said, had been 'indefatigable in doing good'.
Ironically, Grey was to die a few years later of another nineteenth-

century killer, typhus, that he caught while ministering to the poor in the back alleys. Daun moved into new lodgings close by the hospital so that he could keep a constant watch on what was going on there. His next difficulty lay in persuading the sick to enter its doors. With echoes of Berlin and St Petersburg, a rumour spread around town that the body of a woman who died in the hospital was so horribly mangled during a post-mortem that when her coffin was opened at the graveside, the appalled mourners found practically nothing of the corpse was left.

Not a word of this was true, according to Daun. 'Another story, equally current, is that the woman was not dead when the surgeons began to open the body and that she even called out to them to spare her,' related the doctor, at the end of his tether. 'What can one do in such a case? No more dissections shall be made but I fear the mischief is already done ... There are several families in Mill Street of the poorest class afflicted with this melancholy complaint, but they evince the greatest aversion to being moved to the hospital ... and prefer dying in the midst of poverty.'

In the meantime, the local businessmen had not been idle in defending their town and their livelihoods from the outrageous slur that they had a foreign killer disease in their midst. On 11 November, a mob of furious merchants and ship owners packed the Commission Room of Sunderland's grand Exchange building, roaring their anger and denouncing the reports of Asiatic cholera as a 'malicious and wicked falsehood'. They went on to pass a series of resolutions to be sent to the Privy Council. John Spence proposed:

> That ... the town is now in a more healthy state that it has usually been at the present season of the year and ... as to the nature of the disorder which has created unnecessarily so great an excitement in the public mind throughout the kingdom, the same is not Indian cholera, nor of a foreign origin, but that the few cases of sickness and death which have taken place in the town ... have in fact been less in number than generally occur

and have arisen from the description hitherto known as common
bowel complaints which visit every town in the kingdom in the
autumn, aggravated by want and uncleanliness.

John Kidson followed this with the motion: 'That the measures
adopted by His Majesty's Government in requiring the shipping
sailing from Sunderland to perform quarantine and more especially in preventing . . . by a ship of war, all ships and other craft
from leaving or entering the port is perfectly unnecessary and
uncalled for, and more especially when it is considered that the
transit of goods and merchandise of every description and unlim-
ited communication by coaches and other means by land is
permitted [from the town] to every other part of the Kingdom.' On
this last point about travel by land, Mr Kidson had some logic on
his side.

Then in a thrust at poor Kell, who was by now fast becoming a
local hate figure, the meeting deeply regretted 'that any individual,
although actuated by proper and honest motives, should have
given information to His Majesty's Government of the existence of
Indian cholera in Sunderland without having first clearly ascertained the fact, and without the knowledge and sanction of the
principal inhabitants, and hopes that the opinion of this meeting
will prevent in future a conduct calculated to bring such disas-
trous consequences, not only to this town but the country at large.'

Kell had decided not to go to the meeting, and when he learnt
about the crowd's ugly mood, he welcomed his lucky escape from
'the unpleasant consequences which might have resulted towards
me in that tumultuous assembly'. By this time, the army surgeon
had had enough. As he saw it, he had tried to do his duty for the
sake of the town, but from now on he would confine himself to the
job he was paid for: worrying about the health of his troops. He
withdrew behind the walls of the great barracks.

The civilian doctors also felt the wrath of the meeting. In a clear
threat to their pockets, the businessmen voted to publish the names
of those medical gentlemen who had supported the idea of informing

London that the cholera was among them. The meaning was not lost on the doctors: anyone on the blacklist would suddenly find himself very short indeed of wealthy private patients. Consequently, an even more extraordinary event was to follow. That evening the meeting reconvened, and sixteen of the town's doctors stood up before it, one after the other, to deny the information that they had sent to London just days before. Their words read like recantations at a show trial:

Mr Dixon: 'The continental cholera has not been imported into Sunderland and the cases of sickness which have taken place in Sunderland are aggravated English cholera.'

Dr Browne: 'The cases of cholera which have occurred in Sunderland arise from the product of our own soil and entirely among ourselves and has not been imported and is not contagious.'

Mr Croudace: concurs with Dr Brown.

Mr Watson: 'English cholera only has prevailed here.'

Mr White: 'Has not seen a case of Asiatic cholera in Sunderland'.

Mr Ward: 'The disease in Sunderland is not a contagious disease and not more aggravated than the epidemics of the four previous autumns.'

Mr Smithson: 'The Asiatic cholera has not taken place in Sunderland.'

Mr Greene: 'The cholera which has appeared in Sunderland has no foreign origin.'

Mr Ferguson: Dissented from the report forwarded to government by the medical board of this town and does not think we have any Asiatic cholera in this town; and believes we are in a more healthy state with the exception of an epidemic of English cholera than we are generally in this season of the year.

Mr Gregory: Dissented from the proceedings of the medical board of this town from their first commencement. We have no disease in this town which he considers Asiatic cholera or any contagious cholera whatever.

By now the rest of the country was looking on aghast. Worried by the damage being done to the reputation of Sunderland's medical profession, an exhausted Dr Clanny called his colleagues back together for a third time within days and between them they concocted a fudge of a statement, aimed at restoring some of their credibility while at the same time keeping the businessmen sweet. They declared that a disease with every symptom of epidemic cholera was in the town, but there was no reason to suppose it had been imported or was contagious. Rather, it seemed to have arisen from something in the atmosphere that had affected people already weakened by lack of proper food and clothing, or from breathing bad air, or from drunkenness or pre-existing disease. And for good measure, they added, stopping trade would do more harm than good by depriving the poor of their livelihoods and putting families in distress.

This was a statement that Clanny at least could sign with a clear conscience for, unlike Kell, he had never believed cholera to be contagious. He was convinced that the disease – which he called hyperanthraxis because he thought the colour of the patient's skin resembled coal or anthracite – stemmed from an excess of carbon dioxide in the atmosphere, and he slept with his bedroom door ajar to avoid a build-up of the gas.

The medical gentlemen then went on to express their hope that their latest pronouncement would 'remove any misconstructions and false reports which have arisen out of this unpleasant affair' and for good measure, they ended by congratulating their fellow citizens on the otherwise good health of the town.

The Privy Council, completely out of patience with these antics and bombarded almost daily with complaints from Daun and Creagh, responded by drafting in another big gun. Dr David Barry, fresh from the devastation of St Petersburg, was ordered to Sunderland. 'You will immediately institute a careful inquiry for the purpose of removing all doubts as to the nature of the disease existing in that town,' his instructions from the Privy Council ran.

You will communicate with all the medical profession and obtain from them all the information they may be able to afford you. You will state to them that you have been dispatched by His Majesty's Government for the express purpose of making these enquiries, and you will require to be furnished with an accurate statement of all the cases which they may have seen of diarrhoea, common and malignant cholera, with a statement of every new case, and you will require to be personally summoned to such as are of an alarming nature.

The very night that Barry arrived he stumbled upon a case that disturbed him. A mother and two children were lying sick and helpless in a 'miserable habitation' with no food, with one single blanket that they had only just been given, and with a third child lying dead in the room. Such was Barry's influence by now that the Privy Council at once dashed off letters to the Chief Magistrate and the Bishop of Durham demanding an inquiry. On 27 November, Barry wrote again to London, but this time the Privy Council was unable to put the matter he raised so quickly to rights. Barry confirmed that the disease now killing people in Sunderland was identical in every respect to that which had so haunted him in St Petersburg.

By now the town's leading physician, Dr William Reid Clanny, was worn out with work and worry. The sixty-one-year-old consultant had not spared himself – Kell referred admiringly to his 'devoted zeal and anxiety' – yet for his pains he was finding himself almost as vilified as the army surgeon. But while Kell was condemned for irresponsible scaremongering, Clanny was accused of the opposite crime of organising a cover-up. He later wrote about the events, trying to vindicate both the town and himself: 'We met the shock with manly firmness,' he insisted, '. . . though, from unavoidable causes, our success was not what it ought to have been,' adding sadly: 'How far I have deserved the calumnies which in certain quarters have been so lavishly heaped upon me, an enlightened and liberal community will now be enabled to judge.'

By 3 December, seven weeks after cholera first struck, the number of cases in Sunderland stood at over 300, and fourteen new patients were being diagnosed each day. Not one of the soldiers under Kell's care, or their wives or children, was among the casualties, however; the surgeon, acting on his conviction that cholera was contagious, had ordered the barrack gates locked as soon as the disease began to spread and had forbidden the families any contact with the town. But for the rest of the country, the prognosis was grim. The day after Barry identified *cholera morbus* in Sunderland, he and Daun were on their way to Newcastle, ten miles distant, where the mayor had just reported what was believed to be a case of Asiatic cholera, the victim dying in nine hours. On Christmas Day the disease struck at Gateshead, just south of the Tyne, where 'the malignity of the pestilence was truly appalling,' according to the *Lancet*. While Sunderland's businessmen threatened and blustered and its doctors vacillated and lied, the killer had broken loose.

CHAPTER 4

The Surgeon's Apprentice

It is no time to be gathering up your stockings, tying the knees of your breeches, adjusting your neckcloth or hunting for your shoes when half a dozen messengers, one after another, are running breathless to call you to a man that has fallen from a scaffold, to a child suddenly seized with alarming fits, to a person apparently dead and just cut down or taken out of water.

Dissertation on the Duties of Youth Apprenticed to the Medical Profession.
William Chamberlaine, surgeon, 1813

It was a huge and daunting undertaking. He was, after all, only nineteen and he was being asked to shoulder quite alone the responsibility for the lives of scores of men, women and children. But he was also a steady young man, conscientious and clever, with a maturity far beyond his years. This slightly built, painfully shy youth was not everyone's first choice of dinner-party guest, but when life took a serious turn, when wisdom was needed more than wit, and strength of character more than charisma, then John Snow would always be in the front rank of candidates. Now as he packed his belongings in the Newcastle house that had been his home for four long, sometimes difficult years, he could only pray that when he returned it would be with no sense of having failed those desperate families he was being sent to help.

As he brought his bag down ready for the cart, he found his
master, William Hardcastle, standing in the hall with a large box at
his feet. John's heart sank when he saw it was a case of brandy.
Perhaps he should have expected it. All argument was, of course, in
vain: Hardcastle was insistent. The surgeon had little truck with his
young apprentice's hardline views on the evils of drink, any more
than with what he regarded as his ridiculous vegetarianism.
Presumably Hardcastle thought that dealing single-handed with a
cholera epidemic would cause even young John, a keen disciple of
the new temperance movement, to throw his principles to the wind
in favour of prescribing the most trusted remedy of practically
every other medical man in the country. Well if so, Hardcastle
would be proved wrong. The apprentice decided to take the dreadful stuff just to avoid a row but he would bring it back unopened.
Whatever he did for the people of Killingworth Colliery, he was
determined it should not include poisoning them with alcohol.

When Drs Barry and Daun confirmed that cholera had arrived
in Newcastle upon Tyne at the end of November 1831, the city
was a flourishing commercial centre and the second largest port
in the country after London, with a population of well over 40,000.
In a repeat pattern of the events in nearby Sunderland, the disease
struck first and hardest in the poorest quarters where the houses
were old and crammed together in the lanes, and where the overcrowding beggared belief. In the area known as Sandgate on the
quayside, it was common for up to twelve people to be sleeping in
one room, four yards wide. And as with Sunderland, the surrounding
area was coal-mining country, the landscape littered with slag heaps
and with the grim pit communities such as that at Killingworth,
where John Snow was bound. Life in those villages was no rustic
idyll: the conditions were often every inch as cramped and squalid
as they were in the slums of the cities.

Like Snow, Thomas Giordani Wright also left home in his teens
in the 1820s to become an apprentice to a Newcastle doctor, and his
master, like John Snow's, was paid to look after the health of some
of the mining families. Wright described riding out one morning in

1824 to visit a patient at Heaton High Pit, passing the village of Ouseburn on his way:

> Your nose is assailed by a combination of all the odours that can render smell disagreeable. [Vapour from] a steam mill and iron foundry on the one hand and lime kilns on the other, with a tripe shop in the van [front] and a general receptacle for manure at the rear, all lend their aid towards this delectable perfume. Nor do your ears enjoy a greater repose: the combined powers of a dozen or two of hammers upon the melodious tones of steam engine boilers from three forges in close continuity, afford a delicious and harmonious tread, while the unchapelled, crowded burial ground, backed and shaded by a pit heap, rising like a mountain in the distance and flanked by a high row of houses with . . . habiliments hanging from the anything-but-glazed windows, present a picture equally agreeable to the eye.

Cholera spread quickly to these miserable places. By the end of January 1832, most of the towns and villages on Tyneside were infected, while Newcastle itself had had nearly 900 cases. The village of Newburn was a cluster of tiny cottages surrounded by mounds of excrement, whose inhabitants were, hardly surprisingly, 'much addicted to spirit-drinking,' according a local doctor. Newburn lost one-tenth of its population of 550 to cholera, including its vicar.

As one of Newcastle's leading medical men and a popular figure on the social scene, Snow's master, William Hardcastle, held two important posts. He was surgeon-apothecary to the local maternity hospital – or 'lying-in' hospital as it was known – as well as medical attendant to the pit village of Killingworth, five miles out of the city. The epidemic at Killingworth presented Hardcastle with something of a dilemma, for it coincided with his taking on yet another responsibility. The parish authorities had just appointed him to look after the growing number of cholera victims among the city's destitute classes. As Hardcastle saw it, he had little choice but to stay at his post and send his young apprentice off to the pit to deal with the crisis there as best he could.

Apprenticeship to an experienced doctor such as Hardcastle was the traditional route into medicine at the time, particularly for a young man with little money or social standing. And John Snow was certainly that. The oldest of nine children, he was born on 15 March 1813, in York in a house on the banks of the river Ouse, one of the poorer parts of town, where his father, William, worked as a labourer. Despite their humble status, the Snows embodied all of the qualities that would later become known as the Victorian virtues. They were an honest, respectable, God-fearing and industrious family with a bent for self-improvement and a strong sense of social duty. One of John's brothers went on to become a clergyman, another ran a temperance hotel, while two of his sisters opened a school. And the whole family became enthusiastic supporters of the York Temperance Society which John helped set up when he was in his early twenties.

As the lad grew, his father William changed his job from labourer to cart driver and eventually to farmer, buying land outside the city and houses to rent out. In the nineteenth century, this was a quantum leap up the socio-economic ladder but even so, John's wealthy and generous uncle, Charles Empson, a friend of Hardcastle's who later opened a bookshop in Newcastle, may well have helped pay for his medical education. After a basic grounding in the three Rs at a school for working-class children in York, the studious boy who excelled at arithmetic was sent off at the tender age of fourteen to begin his pupillage with Mr Hardcastle, some eighty miles from home.

In the early nineteenth century, the apprentice system was a lottery, with the hapless patients the eventual winners or losers. The cost varied hugely – parents could pay anything from 5s (now £11) to £500 (now £22,000) – and so did the quality of the training. Some boys were treated as little more than drudges by their master's family, working gruelling hours and gaining precious little by way of medical education; and, as John Snow was to do at Killingworth, they also took on responsibilities way beyond their experience. The London surgeon, William Chamberlaine, spelt out the dangers for the unfortunate patient: 'The life of the father of a numerous family, of a beloved wife, of an only child, the fate of a whole family, often depends on an apothecary's apprentice. How often have the most lamentable mistakes occasioned death?' No one was keeping a tally, but a strong suspicion that the answer to Chamberlaine's hypothetical question might well prove to be 'very often indeed', had led the Government, in 1815, to introduce new training requirements for apothecaries, who were on the first rung of the medical hierarchy. Even so, medical education was still to remain chaotic and largely unregulated for decades to come.

James Paget, who later gave his name to a disease of the bone and a condition of the nipple, began his career as an apprentice in 1830 – three years after Snow went to Mr Hardcastle – paying a fee of 100 guineas. Paget and Snow were later to work together. Much of the daily work was tedious, Paget claimed. 'One's time was chiefly occupied in dispensing, seeing a few outpatients of the poorer classes, receiving messages, keeping accounts and, at Christmas time, making out bills and receiving payments,' he recalled.

When Paget's master came in from his rounds each day, he would sit down to dictate the medical notes for each patient he had seen, followed by the prescriptions for his young assistant to make up. 'The pills to be duly rolled and smoothly rounded, and the leeches to be put in their boxes with scarcely any struggling room,' Paget remembered. He also saw most of the outpatients who turned up at the shop, mainly cases of ulcerated legs, coughs and colds, and minor injuries. His duties also included indulging the fancies of the working country people who believed that being bled once or twice a year was good for their health and insisted on undergoing the procedure until they fainted or, at least, became white-faced and weak-kneed. But Paget believed that in his time as an apprentice he learnt nearly as much about anatomy as most

medical students after a year of hospital study, and more about
medical and surgical practice than the students did after two years
in a hospital.

Snow's great friend in later life, Sir Benjamin Ward Richardson,
looked back fondly on his own apprentice days. 'I was taught to
beat opium and soap together to make pills,' he recalled. 'I wrote
fresh labels for all the bottles, and I learned not only the names but
the nature and quality of the medicines, and was soon a scholar in
the mystery as well as in the art. It was not long before I saw
patients on my own account, and once, on Mr Hudson going away,
I was entrusted with the care of those of the outside sick people
who would have me.'

The apprentice was obviously much at the mercy of his master
for his education and general treatment, but there were pitfalls for
the master, too, according to William Chamberlaine: 'When in the
course of a year we see a youth whose parents have with difficulty
been able to raise £50 or £100 as an apprentice fee, dashing away
with a new pair of expensive boots every two or three months, a
massy gold chain and three or four large gold-mounted seals dan-
gling on his watch, which he had not when he first came; when we
hear of his sporting a road horse or a gig every time he is allowed
a holiday . . . it behoves you to look to your till,' he warned. But
Chamberlaine also recommended treating an apprentice with the
respect due to a fledgling member of the professional classes,
although as much for practical reasons as for etiquette: 'It is
degrading to send him to mess with the servants in the kitchen . . .
a practice followed by many evil consequences: bastard children,
marriages with cook-maids and learning gambling from footmen.'

Neither the contents of William Hardcastle's till nor the virtue of
his servants were in the slightest danger from the young John Snow,
whose favourite leisure pursuits were swimming and going for long
country hikes, but there were tensions nonetheless in the
Hardcastle household during the six years of the young man's stay,
mainly, ironically, because of his puritanical lifestyle. In the 1820s,
the temperance movement was a new phenomenon, generally

regarded as the province of a handful of fanatics and cranks. Most people considered alcohol to be highly beneficial to the health, warming and stimulating to the system, and increasing energy and physical strength. For a medical man to decry its use and refuse to prescribe it was seen at best as eccentric and by some doctors and patients as positively negligent.

As a young man, Snow's friend Richardson was famous in his social circle as a connoisseur of wine, not to mention a dab hand at making whisky punch, and if an abstainer came to him for a medical report for life insurance, Richardson would count the man's refusal to take alcohol as a black mark against him. After carrying out a series of experiments in later life, however, Richardson changed his views completely. He concluded that alcohol was a potent drug rather than a nourishing food, and a narcotic not a stimulant. In 1869, he finally became a total abstainer and yet, almost forty years after John Snow had embraced the temperance cause, alcohol was still so well regarded that despite Richardson's by then considerable professional reputation, he found himself shunned by most of his fellow doctors. 'I remember nothing like the mischief which befell me when I made the first sortie [as an abstainer],' he wrote. 'Before then my lecture rooms had been filled with medical men. Afterwards, the rooms were simply vacant . . . I was marked . . . with the sin of disbelief in the ancient faith.'

As John Snow grew up in the 1820s, England's anti-alcohol movement was being born, and it found its greatest support in Lancashire and in Snow's home county of Yorkshire. At the age of seventeen, Snow became an advocate of temperance, or drinking in moderation, but while he was under Hardcastle's roof, he went further, 'taking the pledge' of total abstinence. Overcoming his shyness and his difficulty in getting himself noticed, the zealous young convert addressed a public meeting, attacking the widespread view that, while excessive drinking was clearly to be discouraged, drinking in moderation was good for the health. 'We might as well say that because gambling a little with small sums does not put a man and his family to the risk of starvation and produce all the distress and crime that gambling to

excess does; therefore, gambling in moderation must be a good thing,'
he declared.

And if this were not enough to drive any right-thinking medical
man to drink, Hardcastle and his household had to cope with the
tiresome apprentice's devotion to another much-derided cause.
When John was three years into his apprenticeship, at about the
time that he renounced alcohol completely, he came across a pamphlet by John Frank Newton, a fervent campaigner in another area
of health, morals and diet. Newton believed that man's natural
sustenance was fruit and vegetables, and thought flesh-eating a
perverse custom that caused all manner of ills, bringing about a
'derangement' in the stomach and liver, an 'undue impetus' to the
brain, disorders of the skin and a check on the 'freedom of the
secretions', and an inflammation of the whole system.

'The name of my apothecary is Verlander and he lives at
Knightsbridge,' Newton informed his readers.

> I never in my life had a medicine chest, and from no person but
> Mr Verlander has medicine of any sort been purchased for . . .
> seven persons. Spirits of wine to burn under coffee and a bottle
> to contain them are the only items of charge in this account . . .
> I may be mistaken, but I am persuaded that there is scarcely
> another instance in this never-ending metropolis of three grown
> persons and four young children under nine years of age incur-
> ring an expense of sixpence only for medicine and medical
> attendance in the course of two years.

The Newtons lived on a diet of dried fruit for breakfast, together
with dry or lightly buttered toast or biscuits, washed down with
weak tea with very little milk. For dinner, they had potatoes and
other vegetables and macaroni, followed by a tart or a pudding
made with as few eggs as possible, and also sometimes a dessert.
Sauces were made from stewed onions and walnut pickle. All the
drinking water was distilled, including that used for making tea,
and the family kept a still for the purpose in their back kitchen.

Newton's convictions were on humanitarian as well as health grounds: he referred to the cultivation of the earth as 'implying a certain degree of intellectual progress, unnecessary to him who contents himself with breaking a stick from a tree and demolishing the first poor defenceless animal he meets with it.' And perhaps not surprisingly, he was also strongly in favour of exercise and opposed to alcohol.

Even though Newton had a famous disciple in the poet Shelley, his views were seen as outlandish, perhaps not in the sophisticated Bohemian circles in which Percy Bysshe Shelley moved, but certainly by the more stolid citizens among whom John Snow lived and worked. Benjamin Ward Richardson told how, during a short spell as a medical assistant in the Yorkshire village of Pateley Bridge in the mid-1830s, Snow's vegetarianism had 'puzzled the housewives, shocked the cooks and astonished the children,' although Richardson added that, at Pateley Bridge at least, 'his culinary peculiarities were attended to with great kindliness.'

Whether Snow's convictions were met with kindliness or with hostility, however, they were non-negotiable – for despite his self-effacing manner, even in his teens John Snow was not a negligible or malleable personality. On the contrary, when he believed himself to be in the right, he possessed a quiet but unshakeable determination, both in matters of science and, most particularly, where his personal convictions and conscience were concerned. On these occasions, he was not the slightest perturbed if others found him ridiculous, infuriating or odd. Hardcastle also became annoyed with him for losing good patients by telling them when there was nothing wrong with them and sending them away without treatment, while the young man's diligence got him into trouble with John Watson, a surgeon in Burnopfield village outside Newcastle, for whom he worked briefly between leaving Hardcastle and moving to Pateley Bridge.

Snow told the Burnopfield story many years later. 'When I was a very young man I went for a brief period to assist a gentleman who had a large parochial practice,' he said.

I found his surgery in a very disorderly state and, thinking on my first day with him that I would enhance myself in his opinion by my industry, I set to work as soon as his back was turned to cleanse the Augean stable. I took off my coat, cleared out the drawers, relieved the counter of its unnecessary covering, re-labelled the bottles and got everything as clean as a new pin.

When the doctor returned he was quite taken by storm with the change and commenced to prescribe in his day book. There was a patient who required a blister [poultice], and the worthy doctor . . . put his hand into a drawer to produce one. To his horror, the drawer was cleansed. 'Goodness,' cried he. 'Why, where are all the blisters?' 'The blisters?' I replied. 'The blisters in that drawer? I burnt them all. They were old ones.' 'My good fellow,' was the answer. 'This is the most extravagant act I ever heard of. Such proceedings would ruin a parish doctor. Why, I make all my parochial people return their blisters when they have done with them. One blister is enough for at least half a dozen patients. You must never do such a thing again.'

Whatever William Hardcastle's differences with Snow, however, the surgeon ensured that the young man received a solid grounding in his profession during his six-year apprenticeship. As well as spending time on the more mundane chores, like Paget and Richardson, Hardcastle's pupil was one of the first students to enrol for lectures and demonstrations at the new Newcastle upon Tyne School of Medicine, and he also had the valuable experience of walking the wards of the local infirmary, thanks to Hardcastle's influence in the town.

Meanwhile through the spring and summer, as the nineteen-year-old Snow did what little he could for the stricken Killingworth miners, and as Hardcastle and his colleagues battled to control the epidemic in the city and the outlying villages, cholera was making great strides across the rest of the country. It had arrived just south of Edinburgh in December 1831, after one of its extraordinary leaps of nearly a hundred miles from north-east England. The Scottish capital itself was hit at the end of January, and then, within days, after another sleight of hand, the disease finally showed itself four hundred miles away in London.

At the beginning of February, doctors working in some of the poorest parts of the English capital reported ten highly suspicious cases. Three of the casualties – a coal dredger, a ship-scraper and an unemployed sailor – lived at Rotherhithe on the Thames in south-east London, and three others – a mother and her young daughter and a woman described as being 'of loose character' – at Lime-house, again on the Thames but this time on the north bank of the river. After studying the medical men's reports, the Board of Health announced that to its great regret there was now little doubt that these cases were the genuine article. By the end of the month, the disease was in Westminster and Chelsea, in the very heart of the city, and three months later over 1,300 Londoners were dead. From London, cholera then fanned out steadily and relentlessly until it was in nearly every part of the country, hitting most of the major cities including Hull, Liverpool, Manchester, Oxford, Exeter and Bristol. And just as in Continental Europe, its arrival almost everywhere was greeted with panic and disorder. The trouble was caused partly by people's suspicions that the doctors were using cholera as an excuse for getting their hands on corpses to dissect and partly by their out-rage at the authorities' unceremonious rush to dispose of the bodies.

The aristocratic Charles Cavendish Fulke Greville, secretary to the Privy Council, was revolted by the behaviour of his fellow cit-izens. On 1 April 1832, he noted in his diary: 'I have refrained for a long time from writing down anything about the cholera because the subject is intolerably disgusting to me, and I have been bored past endurance by the perpetual questions of every fool about it. It is not, however, devoid of interest. In the first place, what has happened here proves that the people of this enlightened, reading, thinking, reforming nation are not a whit less barbarous than the serfs in Russia, for precisely the same prejudices have been shown here that were found at St Petersburg and at Berlin.'

There had been some disgraceful scenes in London, Greville said. 'The other day a Mr Pope, head of the cholera hospital in Marylebone, came to the Council Office to complain that a patient who was being removed [to hospital] with his own consent had been taken out of his chair by the mob and carried back, the chair broken, and the bearers and surgeon hardly escaping with their lives ... In short, there is no end to the ... uproar, violence, and brutal ignorance that have gone on, and this on the part of the lower orders, for whose especial benefit all the precautions are taken.' The day before Greville put his account on paper, the London surgeon Joseph Houlton, of Lisson Grove, had written to the Home Secretary, Lord Melbourne, to complain about the treatment meted out to his assistant who was beaten by a mob when visiting a cholera patient. The poor injured young man was then chased home by hundreds of people 'with shouting and disorder,' Houlton said.

And the trouble was by no means confined to the capital. Rioting broke out several times in Liverpool that summer. On one occasion, crowds of men, women and children smashed windows at the Toxteth Park cholera hospital and pelted members of the local board of health with bricks. Then, on 2 September, violence erupted in Manchester when a mob stormed Swan Street Hospital, breaking down the gates, wrecking furniture and fighting a pitched battle with the police. Calm was restored only when the 15th Hussars arrived on the scene. In this case, however, despite the old Etonian Greville's lofty disdain for the foolishness of the lower classes, the crowd had a point. Two days earlier, a local man, John Hare, had gone to Swan Street hoping to see his four-year-old grandson who had just lost both of his parents to cholera. He was refused admission but was told that the boy was getting better. The next day Hare went to the local board of health to enquire again, this time only to be told that the boy was dead. The small body was handed over already in its coffin, and when Hare raised the lid, he found that the boy's head had been removed and replaced by a brick. The culprit turned out to be a young doctor acting on his own initiative, who had smuggled the head out of the hospital in order to dissect it.

The authorities ordered an inquiry and, in the meantime, the doctor responsible was run out of town, but the incident did little to inspire public confidence in the medical profession. The root of the trouble lay in doctors' genuine difficulties in obtaining bodies for the dissections that were – and, to a large extent, still are – an essential part of medical training. Giving evidence before a Parliamentary committee in 1828, the prominent surgeon Sir Astley Cooper – who was created a baronet for removing a sebaceous cyst from George IV's scalp and whose pupils included the poet John Keats – estimated that there were then 700 medical students at the London anatomical schools and that each of them required two bodies for dissection and a third on which to practise surgical procedures. In their subsequent report the MPs noted that demand had forced prices up from between one to two guineas per 'subject' at the end of the eighteenth century to ten or even sixteen guineas.

One of Snow's instructors at the Newcastle School of Medicine, John Fife, later to become Sir John, once dissected the corpse of a hunch-backed maker of surgical instruments, which he had bought for £10 while the man was still alive. When closing the deal, the canny vendor, clearly worried that Fife might prove just a little too keen for comfort, had added the stipulation: 'possession not to be taken until after death'.

The only source of corpses then clearly sanctioned by law and generally accepted by the public was a grim one; namely, the gibbet. The bodies of executed criminals were handed over for public dissection, and this final indignity was regarded as an important part of the punishment, for people believed that, come Resurrection Day, the Almighty would deign to raise only whole, decently buried bodies from the grave. In 1829, the apprentice Thomas Giordiani Wright paid 2s 6d to watch Fife dissect the brain of Jane Jameson, who had been convicted of murdering her mother: 'The poor woman was hung this morning at the old place of execution near the barracks ... The body will, I suppose, be exposed to public gaze for a few days when she will be anatomised by Mr Fife.' Fife did an impressive job, Giordiani reported, partly, he thought, because the surgeon had such a fine fresh specimen on which to work.

Inevitably, supply and demand had given rise to the loathsome and lucrative business of grave-robbing, which, though despised and feared in every stratum of society, was legally something of a grey area. What was clearly not a grey area, however, was the refinement known as 'burking', after the infamous Messrs Burke and Hare. This enterprising pair of so-called 'resurrection men' had come up with a scheme that obviated the tiresome business of creeping out at night under cover of darkness lugging crowbars, spades and sacks; digging up tombstones and coffins with an eye out for the watchman, and then trundling the cumbersome merchandise back through the silent streets. How much easier to lure the goods to some suitable spot while they still breathed and then snuff the life out of them at a convenient moment. In 1828 in Edinburgh, William Burke and William Hare murdered at least sixteen people and sold their bodies to the physician Robert Knox. Hare turned King's evidence in return for a pardon, but Burke was convicted and hanged.

And in London on 5 December 1831, two months before cholera arrived in the capital, the burkers John Bishop and Thomas Williams were hanged at Newgate crossroads near the present site of the Old Bailey before a jeering, cheering crowd of 30,000 people. Their victims had included a fifteen-year-old street boy. In a satisfying piece of rough justice, their bodies then went for dissection – Williams to St Bartholomew's Hospital and Bishop to King's College.

Sir Astley Cooper told the MPs that the resurrectionists were: 'The lowest dregs of degradation; I do not know that I can describe them better. There is no crime they would not commit, and as to myself, if they would imagine I would make a good subject, they really would not have the smallest scruple – if they could do the thing undiscovered – to make a subject of me.'

But it was not only suspicions of burking by the very medical men who were supposed to be caring for them that upset people; the burials were also causing uproar. The Board of Health, still unsure that cholera was contagious but wisely not prepared to take the risk, had issued special instructions for the disposal of victims: 'The bodies ... should on no account be carried into the churches ... Such bodies should, without being washed, be wrapt in the clothes in which they may have died and deposited as soon as possible in a well-fastened coffin, carefully pitched.'

When the authorities in Exeter tried to follow these rules in disposing of two of the city's first casualties, however, they sparked a riot. No sooner had the victims, a husband and wife, drawn their last breaths, than the undertaker slammed them into their coffins, nailed the lids down hard, covered the boxes with tar and wrapped them in brown paper. The man died first, and while his corpse was undergoing this hasty and undignified treatment, his wife lay still conscious in the next room. The news spread fast about what was seen as a shocking indecency, and as the undertakers' men brought the bodies out for burial, they found themselves greeted by a huge angry crowd. The sight of the coffins being carried under-hand rather than shoulder-high in the traditional manner – another measure that was recommended on sanitary grounds – only roused the onlookers to further fury, and they began shouting that the couple were being buried alive or buried like dogs. By the time the rowdy procession arrived at the cemetery, the police had to battle the mob to regain order.

Lurid stories about people being buried alive were given extra power by the fact that muscle contractions occasionally made the bodies twitch after death, causing 'terror to ignorant persons and persons not ignorant,' according to one medical man. A London surgeon called Ward saw this for himself in a twenty-five-year-old patient. 'Ten minutes after he died while I was talking to his bereaved mother, I was quickly summoned by the nurse who told me that my patient was not dead, as she had seen him move,' Ward recounted. 'On my return to his bedside I found him without pulse or respiration. In two or three minutes, however, I was almost as astonished as the nurse had been at seeing the eyes of my dead patient open and move slowly in a downward direction. This was followed by a movement of the right arm, previously lying by his side, across the chest. There was likewise a slight movement of his right leg. The motion of the eyes occurred but once; those of the limbs were repeated to a greater or less degree four or five times, and fully half an hour lapsed before they ceased entirely.'

All the while disease and disorder ran amok through Britain's towns and cities during that spring and summer of 1832, the young John Snow remained at his post at the Killingworth Colliery, coping calmly and uncomplainingly with the epidemic that raged there for weeks. No records exist of his time there but, according to a friend in later life, everyone agreed that he acquitted himself well. Predictably, he worked night and day to try to relieve the suffering of the families in that squalid village, and insofar as anyone was able to do anything for cholera patients in the early nineteenth century, he was considered to have had some success – even without the aid of Hardcastle's brandy, although the surgeon was not best pleased to be told so when he congratulated his trainee on his efforts. The hated case of spirits accompanied the young man back to Newcastle, the bottles still corked. Yet despite Snow's efforts, the churchyard at nearby Longbenton where the Killingworth victims are buried testifies to the ravages of the disease; alongside the neat rows of tombstones which mark the resting places of those who died in an orderly fashion, lie the unmarked graves into which the bodies of the cholera dead were hastily thrown. And while no records have survived of the causes of deaths, the number who died in the parish that year was 235, compared with the usual figure of under a hundred.

Shouldered alone and at such a young age, this was an experience that changed John Snow's life for ever. Years afterwards he recalled how he had watched men struck down as they worked at the coal face being carried up to the surface on the brink of total collapse. But moved to compassion as this quiet and undemonstrative lad was, a detached part of him was also intrigued by this extraordinary disease. How, exactly, did it affect the body? And how was it being spread? Why were some people struck down and not others? Why did so few medical men succumb? Why had he himself emerged unscathed from the midst of so much sickness?

Thirty-two thousand people were to die in the United Kingdom before this epidemic was done. Then strangely and typically, in the Autumn of 1832, a year after it had first appeared, the disease petered out for no reason that anyone could fathom. The panic subsided and the boards of health were wound down. Doctors, politicians, clergymen and the rest of His Majesty's subjects alike breathed a sigh of relief, thanked God for deliverance, and turned their minds to other matters. Cholera was largely forgotten – until the next time. But not for John Snow. Over the months and years to come, as he qualified as a doctor, set himself up in medical practice and carried out research into many other areas of medicine, he would ponder the symptoms of this disease and how it appeared to attack the body; and he also thought about the habits of the Killingworth miners and the conditions in which they and their families lived. And quietly, gradually, he began to get the glimmerings of an idea.

CHAPTER 5

A London Training

To become a successful eye surgeon, a man must be prepared to ruin a whole hat-full of eyes

George James Guthrie, surgeon, Westminster Hospital, 1827–43

In October 1837, when John Snow enrolled at the Westminster Hospital – then in Broad Sanctuary opposite Westminster Abbey – for twelve months' clinical practice, the former military surgeon George Guthrie was one of several trail-blazing surgeons on the staff. Snow's other teachers included Sir Anthony Carlisle, a man who had studied art under Sir Joshua Reynolds and anatomy under John Hunter, the founder of modern surgery. An entertaining fellow, Carlisle included Samuel Coleridge among his many famous friends and had offered to cure the poet of his notorious drug addiction. 'No one tells a story like Carlisle,' remarked the writer Charles Lamb. All in all, it was a very different world from the Newcastle Infirmary, Burnopfield village in Northumbria and the Yorkshire hamlet of Pateley Bridge, which had been the young Snow's experience to date.

Opened in 1719 to treat the sick poor, the Westminster had grown over the years from fewer than twenty beds to close to a hundred by the time Snow arrived, despite an occasionally colourful history. There had been a major scandal in 1827, ten years before John

Snow enrolled, for instance, when a feud broke out between rival factions of doctors. Guthrie had quarrelled with another surgeon, Charles Ferguson Forbes, over the running of the Westminster Eye Infirmary, and Forbes challenged him to a duel. When Guthrie, with uncharacteristic cool, refused, one of his pupils, Frederick Hale Thompson, deliberately insulted Forbes so that he would be called out instead. In a final showdown Thompson and Forbes faced each other with pistols on Clapham Common, where, mercifully, their bravado turned out to be greater than their marksmanship. They both emerged unscathed, despite firing three shots apiece before their seconds intervened. From then on Guthrie's pupil was known as 'bullet-proof Thompson'. It was hardly the sort of atmosphere likely to appeal to a serious-minded young teetotaller from the provinces whose idea of riotous living was a marathon swim down the Tyne or a long hike over the Yorkshire moors. Despite such antics, however, the hospital had a reputation for excellence, and when it came to medical training, walking the wards at the Westminster was held in high esteem.

Snow's stint at the Westminster marked the final stage in his quest to become a doctor. He had arrived in the capital in October 1836 on foot, trudging Dick Whittington-like from York to London, with a detour by way of Bath to visit his uncle. His purpose was to attend a course of lectures and gain London hospital experience, which would allow him to sit the exams of the Society of Apothecaries and also of the Royal College of Surgeons, both of which he needed in order to qualify.

In the first half of the nineteenth century, a man calling himself a doctor might hold any one of a bewildering range of qualifications, from a university degree – which required the study of classical Greek and Latin medical texts – to one of the medical licences issued by a plethora of different authorities including, bizarrely, the Archbishop of Canterbury; or he might have absolutely no qualifications or even any medical training at all. Unsurprisingly, this chaotic situation had resulted in huge anomalies; for instance, while grocers were free to peddle any home-made remedies they chose, a member of the Royal College of Physicians of London with a medical degree from Oxford or Cambridge could be disciplined for dispensing drugs, due to the college's wish to keep its distance from the druggists and the apothecaries.

Sir Henry Halford, the royal courtier who had presided over the first Board of Health in 1831, held the then conventional view among the medical elite that the study of the classics was an essential part of medical education, describing the texts as: 'Those depositories of the wisdom of ancient days, which allure all men that are studious into that delicate and polished kind of learning.' Sir Henry urged medical students to pore over the literature night and day, with the happy result that: 'If the study of the classics be directed with judgement, it will be found that they exhibit the best models of order and of taste . . . Classical knowledge will be applicable on 10,000 occasions to illustrate and adorn science.' But Sir Henry was a physician, one of that exclusive band at the pinnacle of the medical hierarchy who never sullied their hands with the messy business of surgery, nor even deigned to touch their patients if they could possibly help it. A hard-pressed apothecary-surgeon, spending his days lancing boils, dressing ulcers, setting bones and draining blood, might have taken issue with the royal doctor about the relevance of 'that delicate and polished kind of learning' to day-to-day medicine as it was practised. Characteristically, Sir Henry whiled away his retirement in the writing of Latin poetry.

John Snow, typically, was following one of the respectable routes into medicine, working his way up the hierarchy from apothecary to surgeon – which his master Hardcastle had been – before eventually going on to eclipse Hardcastle by achieving Sir Henry's status, that of physician. For his lectures, Snow enrolled at the private Hunterian School in Great Windmill Street, Soho, founded in 1769 by William Hunter, famous in his own right, but also the brother of John Hunter, the founder of modern surgery. Here he studied anatomy and physiology, surgery, medicine, *materia medica* (pharmacology), chemistry, botany, midwifery and medical jurisprudence. *Punch* magazine was not convinced about the usefulness of all of these subjects: 'The knowledge of the natural class and order of a buttercup must be of the greatest service to a practitioner in treating a case of typhus fever or ruptured blood vessel. At some of the Continental hospitals the pupil's time is wasted at the bedside of the patient, from which he can get only practical information. How much better is the primrose-investigating curriculum of study observed at our own medical schools.' James Paget concluded, however, that while the knowledge he gained from studying botany was largely useless, the discipline of acquiring it was 'beyond all price'.

It was at the Hunterian that Snow met a fellow student called Joshua Parsons. Although Parsons teased him about his vegetarianism which he thought bad for the health, the two became firm friends. The life of a typical medical student of the time consisted of steeplechases in the dissection room, cheating in the Latin exams, flirting with barmaids, and gin and water until three o'clock in the morning, according to *Punch* magazine. And the students' reputation for wildness and black humour knew no bounds after one of their number at the Great Windmill School nearly caused a riot by climbing onto the roof and dropping a severed leg down the chimney of the house next door. The blood-spattered limb fell into a cooking pot where a housewife was boiling up a stew. The woman ran screaming into the street, and the young man escaped being lynched on the spot only when his friends bribed the crowd into handing him over.

All this was a far cry from the innocent world of Snow and Parsons. They met through their mutual habit of working late into the night in the dissecting room and then shared lodgings in Bateman's Buildings, a row of cheap boarding houses in Soho, a few minutes' walk from the Hunterian. It was hardly a good address, but their accommodation was probably no worse than this description of typical medical students' rooms of the time:

The landlady and the furniture had both seen better days, as landladies and furniture generally have. The bed curtains were of dark, glazed calico, to keep clean a long time and not show the dirt when they ceased to be so. The dingy walls were redolent of tobacco, and there was in the sitting room a dark, old-fashioned mahogany table whereon was to be seen ... sundry circles of evaporated moisture somewhat about the circumference of the bottom of a quarter pot. The pattern of the carpet had long been obliterated ... the looking glass had been scored all to pieces ... and a few pictures of that kind only met with in lodging houses and pawnbrokers' shops adorned the walls.

Any tobacco film on the walls or ale stains on the tables at Bateman's Buildings certainly grew no worse during the tenancy of John Snow and Joshua Parsons, however, for the two young men lived a studious and frugal life, shunning the temptations of the city around them. When not cutting up corpses or poring over text books, they spent their time competing in trials of strength, trying to settle once and for all their argument about whether vegetarianism was good for the constitution. Parsons considered he had won when, at the end of a fifty-mile hike to St Albans and back one Bank Holiday Monday, Snow was forced to take an omnibus in the Edgware Road for the last leg of the journey.

In fact, though, beneath his jokey exterior, Parsons worried that Snow's refusal to eat meat was having a serious effect on his health. He noticed that his friend suffered from bouts of exhaustion that sometimes prevented him from finishing his day's studies. And he also remarked that the smallest cut or graze would sometimes make Snow's face flush bright red, his temperature shoot up alarmingly and his pulse race, and he wondered if this were not due at least in part to his frugal diet. On one such occasion Parsons seriously considered sending for Snow's uncle, Charles Empson.

Even so, Parsons himself was unwittingly responsible for some further damage to Snow's health. By the time Snow took up his studies at the Hunterian, he had been a vegetarian for nearly eight years, and he used to say that the diet suited him admirably provided he supplemented it with butter, milk and eggs. One morning at breakfast, however, Parsons, who could never resist an opportunity to tease people, asked his friend what vegetable he was currently eating. 'The joke went home; and the use of milk as a food for a pure vegetarian became too absurd for consistency,' Richardson recounted. 'The milk, therefore, must be put aside, and the butter and the eggs.' It was hardly surprising, given that no one then understood how to ensure that even a vegetarian, let alone a vegan, diet was properly balanced, that Snow paid the price of his principled stand. 'The experiment did not answer; the health of our pure vegetarian gave way under the ordeal,' said Richardson.

Throughout his life, Snow continued to argue in favour of a diet rich in vegetables and low in alcohol, but with his usual honesty he admitted that in his case taking his views to extremes had caused problems, and in later life he followed his friends' advice by taking the occasional piece of meat and glass of wine. His constitution was never strong. As a young man he suffered a bout of what was diagnosed as phthisis pulmonalis – a wasting condition that was probably pulmonary tuberculosis – but he recovered with the help of plenty of fresh air. Then, in 1845, he went down with acute kidney problems, and was forced to take a break from his strict schedule of work and research. He recuperated by going to stay with Parsons who by then had moved to a quiet country practice.

While they were at Bateman's Buildings, Parsons noted personal qualities in his friend that characterised him throughout his life. Joshua described Snow as not especially brilliant or original in his thinking, although later events were to prove Parsons quite wrong about this. What distinguished Snow from all the rest, in Parsons' view, was his tireless determination to pursue every scientific investigation relentlessly to its logical conclusion. There were no short-cuts, no leaps of faith and no unquestioning acceptance of untested traditional wisdom, but organised procedure, sound experiment and careful observation. This step-by-step approach, which seems to have come naturally to Snow, was in fact a precursor of the modern method that is now the basis of all medical research.

And Parsons also saw in Snow a selflessness and decency that seems to have struck everyone who met him. Neither money nor fame held any attractions for Snow and, as Parsons observed, his sole aim in all his work was the advance of medicine: 'The object of this steady pursuit with him was always truth. The naked truth for its own sake was what he sought and loved. No consideration of honour or profit seemed to have the power to buy his opinions on any subject.'

At the Hunterian, Snow carried out his first recorded piece of research. His chemistry lecturer, Dr Hunter Lane, read about the practice of injecting dead bodies with arsenic to preserve them for dissection and asked Snow to try it. The procedure seemed to work well and was used on two or three other bodies, but in the middle of dissecting one of the corpses, a student was taken violently ill with stomach cramps, vomiting and diarrhoea – the typical symptoms of arsenic poisoning. Later, again during a dissection, five more students became sick with bowel complaints. Snow noticed that the corpse in question 'gave out a peculiar colour which I suspected arose from an arsenic rising in combination from the volatile products of decomposition'.

To test his idea that the body was giving off arsenic, he took some samples, put them aside and then examined them carefully a few weeks later. The tissues had been drenched in arsenic, but now no trace of the poison remained. He followed this up by leaving some rotting animal flesh on a dish with arsenic, and putting a bell jar over the top to collect the gasses given off. After a couple of weeks, he added hydrogen to the air in the jar to make it flammable and burnt it, using a small jet and holding a piece of glass in the flame. Left behind on the glass after the air had burnt off was a small quantity of metallic arsenic. He had proved his theory – the students were being gassed by arsenic fumes. 'I expressed my conviction that this mode of injection was dangerous,' Snow wrote, 'and it was discontinued at the school.'

Snow passed the Royal College of Surgeons' exams in May 1838 and those of the Society of Apothecaries in October. He asked permission to sit the latter exam in July because he wanted to apply for a vacancy as an apothecary at the Westminster Hospital. But despite excellent references from William Hardcastle, two Yorkshire doctors and several London lecturers, including Mr Anthony White and Sir Anthony Carlisle, the Apothecaries stood firm and refused to take into account his hospital experience in Newcastle. They made him wait until October, losing him the chance of a post that would have given him an excellent footing on the ladder to private practice and a good living.

Richardson claimed the Apothecaries had agreed to such requests in the past, and blamed this refusal on Snow's humble background and lack of powerful friends. When he was turned down the first time, Snow wrote again, asking for leniency and expressing his confidence in the Apothecaries' kindness, Richardson said, adding: 'The confidence was misplaced. The Blackfriars Shylocks demanded their pound of flesh.'

The *Lancet*'s editor Thomas Wakley was no fan of the Worshipful Company of Apothecaries either. He described what a young man could expect on turning up for his examination at Apothecaries Hall – or Rhubarb Hall, as Wakley dubbed it: 'The guide has conducted the candidate into a large room in which, if after-dinner cups have not prevented, twelve examiners are found dispersed at four tables . . . It is quite a matter of accident, a lottery, whether the candidate is examined by a pert puppy or an empty-headed bully, by a self-satisfied sneer or a superficial professor who has, at any rate, a due sense of the proprieties of life and might behave like a gentleman.'

Gentlemanly or not, Snow's examiners – who made it quite clear that they hadn't forgotten the matter of the job at the Westminster – nevertheless had the decency to pass him. Not everyone was so fortunate or so philosophical in their dealings with the Worshipful Company. A few months earlier, a young man had been brought before the magistrates for setting about the tenants of Rhubarb Hall with a bludgeon after they had had the temerity to fail him.

Snow's contemporary James Paget took the Royal College of Surgeons' exams at the same time as Snow, and described how ten examiners sat at a long curved table, each taking a candidate in turn. Paget's chief examiner was Anthony White, a protégé of Sir Anthony Carlisle at the Westminster, and one of the most popular teachers. Paget found White's questions easy and then managed to impress the panel by a bit of a fluke: 'I brought them to a close by giving an account of the otic ganglion and its nerve communications in reply to some enquiry about branches of the fifth nerve. That ganglion was then known to few and he who knew about it seemed to be thought sure to know all common things.'

After Mr White, Sir Astley Cooper, who had given evidence to Parliament about body-snatching, asked a few questions. Again, Paget's luck was in: 'He seemed satisfied, though I did not answer them well,' Paget modestly recalled, 'and then I was courteously dismissed and Sir Astley claimed acquaintance with my father – thought erroneously he had fought him when they were boys together in Yarmouth – and asked me to breakfast.' Snow's family connections didn't merit an invitation to breakfast with the likes of Sir Astley, nevertheless, along with Paget he too passed the exams of the Royal College of Surgeons.

CHAPTER 6

A Very Peculiar Man

He took no wine nor strong drink; he lived on anchorite's fare, clothed plainly, kept no company, and found every amusement in his science books, his experiments and simple exercise

Sir Benjamin Ward Richardson on John Snow

In December 1846, the American mail ship, the SS Arcadia, docked in Liverpool carrying momentous news. The surgeon Jacob Bigelow had written to a London friend about an amazing demonstration he had just watched at Massachusetts General Hospital in Boston. A dentist called William Morton had rendered a certain Gilbert Abbot unconscious using a sponge soaked in ether and a glass inhaler, while the surgeon John Warren removed a tumour from his jaw. When he woke up, Abbot told the astounded spectators that he had felt nothing.

The story spread fast. Was this the longed-for breakthrough that would finally drag surgery out of the Dark Ages? On 21 December at University College Hospital, London, Robert Liston amputated the leg of a butler called Frederick Churchill while a student administered ether. With his legendary speed, Liston did the job in an extraordinary twenty-six seconds but, with the subject blissfully unconscious, a surgeon could now take his time over tricky procedures without having to worry about prolonging the patient's agony. Like all surgeons of his day, Liston had had his fair share of both horror and farce. On one occasion, he had been in the middle of removing a bladder stone when his panic-stricken patient broke loose, ran out of the room and down the hall and locked himself in a lavatory. Hot on his heels, Liston broke down the door and dragged the screaming man back to the operating table.

Another patient told the anaethesia pioneer, James Simpson, how it felt to be awaiting surgery in those days: 'A patient preparing for an operation was like a condemned criminal preparing for execution,' the man explained. 'He counted the days till the appointed day came. He counted the hours of that day. He listened for the echo in the street of the surgeon's carriage. He watched for his step in the room, for the production of his dreaded instruments . . . And then he surrendured his liberty to the cruel knife.'

Down the ages, surgeons had drugged patients with plants like marijuana or mandragora (mandrake). 'Give me to drink mandragora . . . That I might sleep out this great gap of time my Antony is away,' says Shakespeare's Cleopatra. They also tried hypnosis and the rather less scientific approach of knocking people out with a punch on the jaw. Nothing was up to the job. By 1840, opium and alcohol were the only remedies considered any use at all, but the massive doses needed caused bad side-effects and sometimes even death.

The highly sophisticated modern specialism of anaesthesiology dates from 1799 when Humphry Davy, the inventor of the miner's lamp, first discovered the properties of nitrous oxide. This compound of nitrogen and oxygen – dubbed laughing gas because patients experience a huge 'high' before unconsciousness sets in – later became popular for pulling teeth, but its short-lived effects made it unsuitable for long operations. In 1805, however, a German apothecary's assistant called Friedrich Serturner extracted the active ingredient in opium and named it morphine, while in 1815 the chemist and physicist Michael Faraday found that ether produced similar effects to nitrous oxide. But not until the 1840s did the real potential of all these substances begin to be exploited in the cause of surgery.

While the use of ether in surgery was revolutionary in the mid-nineteenth century, the preparation itself – a distillation of sulphuric acid and alcohol – had been discovered as long ago as the thirteenth century by the Spanish chemist Raymundus Lullius, who named it sweet vitriol. It was another 300 years before the Swiss alchemist Paracelsus discovered its sleep-inducing powers.

Snow was fascinated by ether. By the time the news broke, he was already interested in the respiratory system, had carried out many experiments on respiration and asphyxia and had written a paper on a new air-pump to be used for the purpose of artificial respiration. Now he started a series of experiments into the effects of different gases in a quest for the perfect anaesthetic that was to last for the rest of his life.

Since the autumn of 1838 when he qualified as a doctor, Snow had spent much of his time in research and study while he waited for paying patients. He had also moved from Bateman's Buildings to better lodgings in nearby Frith Street, off Soho Square, where he 'nailed up his colours', as he put it, as a medical man. He was to go on to obtain his Bachelor of Medicine degree from the University of London and the following year his MD, or doctorate, which meant that he had reached the status of physician, overtaking his master William Hardcastle and many of his instructors at the Hunterian and the Westminster. He would have achieved his goal fifteen years earlier had he been able to afford to go to university. Snow eventually became a licenciate of the Royal College of Physicians, the highest rank that was open to him; only those with degrees from Oxford or Cambridge could attain the status of Fellow of the RCP.

Staying on in the capital was a tough option. Most students who came to London to finish their training went straight back to the provinces once they had qualified, where it was far easier to earn a living. Joshua Parsons, for example, Snow's friend from Bateman's Buildings, became a country practitioner in Somerset. Earning a decent income depended on attracting wealthy private patients, and the competition in the capital was huge. John Snow had no rich, powerful friends to push him on his way.

His reputation was helped, though, through joining the famous Westminster Medical Society, which had a tradition of encouraging young doctors. The society – whose members had been so taken aback in 1830 at the Russian prize for the best work on cholera – met weekly to read research papers, watch demonstrations of new devices and, most of all, to discuss their ideas. Snow said that the 'Westminster Medical', as it was known, played a crucial part in his being able to stay on in London.

Even so, his shyness and rather husky voice which put him at a disadvantage as a speaker, meant that he took a long time to be accepted. At first everyone completely ignored him. Then at last someone deigned to refer to him as the 'last speaker', but it was many months before anyone used his name or spoke up to support his views. With his usual quiet determination, however, Snow was neither offended nor deterred. And as usual with him, his persistence was eventually rewarded: in 1855 the members of the Medical Society of London, as the 'Westminster Medical' was then called, elected as their president the man they had shunned when he first tried to take part in their debates.

Despite the overnight sensation that ether had caused, surgeons were initially wary of using it on a routine basis because of confusion over its administration: no one knew what the correct dose should be or how to ensure that a patient received it. Snow identified the key problems immediately. The greatest skill, he said, lay in knowing how much ether the patient had been given, and in monitoring his ether status at all stages during the operation. This meant that the anaesthetist had to know the strength of the vapour he was administering, which, in turn, required a suitable apparatus for the purpose; otherwise, it was impossible to know, let alone to regulate, the precise mix of air and ether the patient was breathing. In fact, Snow found that controlling the concentration of ether turned out to be relatively simple: it depended first on the temperature of the gas and, second, on using an inhaler capable of regulating the flow. With his customary methodic approach, he set about designing an inhaler that would meet his requirements. The resulting apparatus consisted largely of a metal water-bath to keep the ether at the correct temperature; an ether chamber; tubes down which the gas could pass, and a face mask with a valve. Snow presented it at a meeting of the Westminster Medical in January 1847.

Snow also embarked on a series of experiments both on animals and on himself to find the safest, most effective concentration of the gas for a given body weight. His friends warned him about the risks he was taking, but Snow saw it as his firm duty to test the gas first on himself before using it on anyone else. And he took what was then a most enlightened view of animal experiments. 'While he held it as a necessity to use inferior animals for the purpose of experiment, he never touched a living thing with the physiologist's finger without having before him some definite object; and never performed experiment on any animal without providing with scrupulous care against the infliction of all unnecessary suffering,' Richardson explained, adding: 'The interests of humanity were, he thought, best advanced by the universal practice of humanity.'

Over the years to come, Snow carried out a long series of experiments on the effects on the body of inhaling different substances, including carbonic acid, carbonic oxide, cyanogen, hydrocyanic acid, ammonia, nitrogen, amylovinic ether, cyanide of ethyle and chloride of amyl. He was looking for the perfect narcotic vapour; effective, easy to administer and completely safe. With his usual order and method, he would first establish the boiling-point of the substance in question and then the point of saturation of air with the vapour at different temperatures. Next he would look at the effects on small animals of inhaling that particular vapour, and determine what concentration of vapour was needed over what period of time in order to produce unconciousness. When he found a gas that would render an animal insensible without any ill effects, he went on to study how much would constitute a fatal overdose – both by means of a quick, large dose, and also a small dose over a long period – and, finally, he would do a post-mortem to discover whether that fatality had resulted from heart failure or respiratory failure. If, after this, the substance still looked promising, he would try it on himself.

Just as Snow was perfecting the technique of administering ether, an incident occurred that gave him an idea of how he might earn a steady living in London. As he came out of one of the hospitals one day, he saw a druggist he knew hurrying along with a large ether apparatus under his arm. 'Good morning to you, doctor,' said his friend, 'but don't detain me, I am giving ether here and there and everywhere, and am getting quite into an ether practice. Good morning, doctor!' And he scurried off. Snow was intrigued, not least because the man concerned knew absolutely nothing about physiology. He lost no time in taking his own superior inhaler along to St George's Hospital to ask to be allowed to administer ether to dental out-patients, and he was soon in regular demand there. The results so impressed one medical man that he mentioned Snow to Mr Cutler, one of the hospital surgeons who was refusing to use ether because he was dubious about the way it was being administered. Within no time, Snow was giving ether on operating days, both at St George's and also at University College Hospital, where Robert Liston took him under his wing. Soon other institutions took him on, including the Hospital for Consumption – now the famous Royal Brompton in Chelsea – and the wonderfully named Hospital for Decayed Gentlewomen, as well as the work-house infirmary in Poland Street, Soho, which was later to play another, very different, role in Snow's life.

In 1847, Snow published a small textbook, *On the Inhalation of the Vapour Ether in Surgical Operations*, which was to become a classic. Here he wrote up his observations of patients before, during and after anaesthesia in nearly eighty operations at St George's and University College, along with tables for calculating the optimum dose of the gas. 'The patients to whom I have given it have been of all ages, from early childhood to nearly eighty years; six of them being upwards of seventy,' he wrote. 'They have been

in the most different states of general health; two or three had
tubercles in the lungs; one had extensive disease of the heart; two
or three had been subject to attacks of conjestion of the head, and
yet there have been no ill consequences from the ether in any case.'

In the course of this work, he discovered that he could keep
patients pain-free for well over an hour with no ill effects if he
allowed them to regain partial consciousness from time to time. He
once kept an elderly man oblivious in this way for two-and-a-half
hours after Liston had applied a thick caustic paste of chloride of
zinc to his face in order to 'burn off' an ulcerating tumour.

Soon after the publication of *On the Inhalation of the Vapour
Ether*, however, another huge discovery eclipsed the use of ether.
James Simpson, an Edinburgh obstetrician, had trained under Liston,
but he had nearly given up medicine in his teens after witnessing a hor-
rendous mastectomy operation on a poor Highland woman. Despite
Liston's skill, it was, he said, like watching torture. Simpson, however,
decided to stay on in the profession in order to dedicate himself to the
conquest of pain. He had been experimenting with many different
sleep-inducing substances with varying degrees of success and at least
one brush with near disaster. One of his servants noticed that choloric
ether mixed with fizzy water looked just like champagne and offered
a glass to the cook. When she dropped unconscious to the floor, the
terrified man rushed into the dining room shouting: 'For God's sake
sir come quick. I've pushioned the cook.'

Nothing could have been in greater contrast to Snow's solitary
studies than Simpson's noisy, convivial pursuit of scientific truth. His
daughter referred to his research sessions as 'anaesthetic seances', but
perhaps wine tasting would be a closer analogy, as Simpson and his
friends gathered round the dining table each night to sample the
evening's selection. Simpson's friend Professor Miller described the
scene: 'Each "operator" having been provided with a tumbler, finger-
glass, saucer, or some such vessel, about a teaspoonful of the respirable
substance was put in the bottom of it. Holding the mouth and nostrils
over the vessel's orifice, inhalation was proceeded with, slowly and
deliberately, all inhaling at the same time, and each noting the effects

as they advanced.' Miller frequently turned up at Simpson's house for breakfast, just to check, he joked, that they were all still alive.

One November night after an exhausting day's work, Drs Simpson, Keith and Duncan sat down at the table as usual and proceeded to sniff substances but with no results until Simpson remembered a heavy, unlikely looking liquid that he had put to one side. He finally discovered it under a pile of wastepaper. Miller described what happened when the trio took their first whiff of chloroform: 'Immediately an unwonted hilarity seized the party; they became bright-eyed, very happy and very loquacious . . . The conversation was of unusual intelligence and quite charmed the listeners.' But in the next minute, those listeners were suddenly jolted out of their pleasant mood by a loud crash, as Simpson, in his own words, found himself 'under the mahogany in a trice, to my wife's consternation and alarm'. Dr Duncan, in the meantime, had slid under his chair with his jaw hanging open, his eyes staring, his head bent half under his body and snoring 'in the most determined and alarming manner,' said Miller. Then there was more noise, and the now horrified spectators looked on as Dr Keith, in a manic state, tried to kick over the supper table and smash everything on it.

Yet almost as fast as they had reacted to the new vapour, the three intrepid researchers began to recover their senses, and the evening then turned into something of a chloroform party, with Mrs Simpson's niece, Agnes Petrie, imagining herself when under the influence in the role of an angel. Simpson was later to enlist Miss Petrie's help in reassuring nervous patients that the drug produced not just a harmless but a positively beatific state of unconsciousness. In the meantime, Dr Keith, who, far from being beatific had returned to his aggressive fixation with the furniture, insisted that he was engaged to dance with the sideboard and tried to drag the massive object into the middle of the floor. The over-excited household finally retired to bed at 3 a.m., miraculously with no lasting damage either to themselves or to the Simpsons' goods and chattels. It was not the sort of soirée that the tenant of 54 Frith Street would have hosted.

*

A clear, colourless liquid, chloroform is more powerful, easier to administer and pleasanter to inhale than ether but also more dangerous, although this wasn't realised at first. Simpson gave it to women in childbirth by sprinkling it on a handkerchief and placing it over their mouth and nose. One of his patients was so delighted with the results that she named her child Anaesthesia. Not everyone was so happy, however. Some religious critics opposed anaesthesia on the grounds that human suffering was a punishment from God, and to take it away was to subvert the Divine Purpose. In particular, there was a row about painless childbirth because in the Genesis story, God's curse upon Eve includes the words: 'In sorrow thou shalt bring forth children.' To ignore this edict was to go against the expressed wishes of the Almighty, it was argued. But Simpson, although a devout Christian, would have none of it. He had done his homework and insisted that elsewhere in the Bible the Hebrew word translated as 'sorrow' in the Adam and Eve passage, was taken to mean effort, toil or labour. Nowhere, he said, was it translated as physical pain. He made his views known in his usual colourful style in a letter to a medical friend: 'By the by, Imloch tells me Dr P. is to enlighten your medical society about the "morality" of the practice [of using chloroform],' he wrote. 'I have a great itching to run up and pound him. When is the meeting? The true moral question is, is a practitioner justified by any principles of humanity in not using it? I believe every operation without it is just a piece of the most deliberate and cold-blooded cruelty.'

John Snow agreed wholeheartedly with the view that chloroform was a boon rather than a blasphemy, although he would have chosen more temperate language with which to make his case. At once, he switched his attention to this new method of pain relief and was soon administering it at St George's and University College. He was also called in to visit wealthy patients at their homes and in hotels, where surgeons commonly operated at that time, working with James Paget, who had passed the Royal College of Surgeon's exams at the same sitting as Snow and was now at St Bartholomew's Hospital, and with Charles Guthrie, son of George

Guthrie who had taught Snow surgery at the Westminster. During the 1850s, Snow kept detailed records of his anaesthesia patients, and they show the variety of his practice. For example, on 4 July 1852 he is found administering chloroform at King's College Hospital to a baby of just eight days, while the surgeon William Fergusson tried to correct the infant's hare lip. Sadly, the face mask proved too big, and the anaesthetic had little effect on the child. The following month he was anaesthetising eighty-seven-year-old Mrs Vallance at her home in Davies Street, while Mr White Cooper operated on a cataract.

The case books also show the range of different procedures, some of them major, that surgeons routinely carried out at locations all over London. Snow records Fergusson excising a breast tumour weighing between three and four pounds from a forty-eight-year-old nurse in Barnes; Paget removing a massive twelve-pound growth from the lower back and buttocks of a young woman at a house in Cavendish Square; Paget amputating part of a Captain Hayes's hand at the patient's home near Hyde Park; and Charles Guthrie and a Dr Chowne carrying out a vaginal examination under chloroform on a newly married woman at Woods Hotel. She had 'suffered great pain during every attempt at coition,' Snow wrote, and the doctors found that her cervix was elongated and enlarged. What was thought to be the cause of the abnormality, and what, if anything, the doctors were able to do for this unfortunate young woman and her husband, Snow does not say.

Although by now he was frequently attending patients at the top of the social scale, Snow continued to offer his services to some of the very poorest. One morning in November, for example, he was giving pain relief to a Mrs Field from the slums of Lower Marsh, Lambeth, during childbirth, while in the afternoon he was to be found administering chloroform to Lady Hood's twelve-year-old son while Mr Rogers removed three molars from the young master's jaw. Two days later, he was back at King's College Hospital with Mr Fergusson, this time as the surgeon operated on an elderly chimney sweep with cancer of the scrotum.

On 24 March, 1853, the usually meticulous John Snow made a slip of the pen when writing up his case notes. The entry for a Mrs Rothery, who had chloroform for the removal of an intractable placenta, gives the patient's address as Buckingham Palace instead of Buckingham Gate. The mistake was not as random as it might at first seem, and it showed that even the unflappable Dr Snow was capable of the odd nervous lapse of concentration. Three years earlier, the royal doctors had asked his advice about administering chloroform to Queen Victoria at the birth of Prince Arthur. Now, with the queen's next child, her eighth, due the following month, Dr Snow had been invited to the palace to give the anaesthetic personally to Her Majesty.

Two weeks later, on Thursday, 7 April, the queen went into labour. Her obstetrician, Dr Locock, was sent for at 9 a.m.. Snow takes up the story:

> I received a note from Sir James Clark [physician in ordinary to Her Majesty] a little after 10, asking me to go to the Palace. I remained in an apartment near that of the Queen, along with Sir James Clark, Dr Ferguson and, for the most part of the time, Dr Locock, till a little after 12. At 12.20 p.m., I commenced to give a little chloroform with each pain by pouring about 15 minims [0.9 millilitres] by measure on a folded handkerchief. The first stage of labour was nearly over when the chloroform commenced.
>
> Her Majesty expressed great relief from the application, the pains being very trifling during the uterine contractions, whilst between the periods of contraction there was complete ease. The effect of the chloroform was not at any time carried to the extent of quite removing consciousness. Dr Locock thought that the chloroform prolonged the intervals between the pains and retarded the labour somewhat. The infant [Prince Leopold] was born at 1.13 p.m., [so] the chloroform [had been] inhaled for 53 minutes. The placenta was expelled in a few minutes, and the Queen appeared very cheerful and well, expressing herself much gratified with the effect of the chloroform.

While he was waiting to be summoned to the queen's bedside, Snow was presented to Prince Albert who, with his unaffected manners, deep sense of honour and fascination with all the latest developments of the modern world, must have been a man after the doctor's own heart. According to Richardson, Snow 'returned much pleased with the Prince's kindness and great intelligence on the scientific points which had formed the subject of their conversation.'

The news that the queen had resorted to pain relief was greeted with both grief and delight in the country. The religious hard-liners shook their heads over Her Majesty's lapse from grace, but the anaesthesia lobby welcomed this celebrity endorsement of their cause, and before long 'anaesthesia à la Reine' was all the rage.

For Snow personally, the trip to the palace had clearly been a success, and it was not surprising that three years later, when the queen was about to give birth to her ninth child, Princess Beatrice, he again received the call. This time, however, the royal labour proved more of an ordeal, and Her Majesty began demanding more pain relief than Snow felt it safe or expedient to provide. In managing this particular birth, the doctors had a difficult balancing act. They were clearly worried about the slow progress of the labour, and Locock gave the queen ergot in order to strengthen her contractions. Ergot is the common name for a fungus, *Claviceps purpurea*, which grows on rye, and which, when taken in sufficient quantities can produce the strange disease known as St Anthony's Fire. In the nineteenth century, ergot was commonly used to induce labour, although an overdose could, and sometimes did, cause the uterus to burst under the strain, killing both mother and child. A safe form of the active ingredient, ergometrine, is still used today. Increasing the queen's contractions also meant increasing her pain, of course; yet at the same time, once in the second stage of labour, Her Majesty must not be too drugged to push.

'The labour occurred about a fortnight later than was expected,' Snow wrote.

It commenced about 2 a.m., when the medical men were sent for. The labour was lingering and, a little after 10, Dr Locock administered half a drachm [half a teaspoonful] of powdered ergot, which produced some effect in increasing the pains. At 11 o'clock, I began to administer chloroform. Prince Albert had previously administered a very little chloroform on a handkerchief . . . for each pain. Her Majesty expressed great relief from the vapour.

Another dose of ergot was given about 12 o'clock and the pains increased somewhat . . . The Queen at this time kept asking for more chloroform and complaining that it did not remove the pain. She slept, however, sometimes, between the pains. Before one o'clock, the head was resting on the perineum, and Dr Locock wished the patient to make a bearing down effect . . . The Queen, however, when not unconscious of what was said, complained that she could not make an effort. The chloroform was left off for three or four pains, and the royal patient made an effort which expelled the head, a little chloroform being given just as the head passed. There was an interval of several minutes before the child was entirely born; it, however, cried in the meantime . . . The Queen's recovery was very favourable.

Not surprisingly, Snow's other patients were avid for hot gossip from the royal bedchamber, but if they expected indiscretions, they had come to the wrong man. Maddeningly, when questioned the doctor would only say: 'Her Majesty is a model patient.' When one woman insisted that she would take no more anaesthetic until Snow had told her, word for word, what the queen had said while she was taking it, Snow replied: 'Her Majesty asked no questions until she had breathed very much longer than you have; and if you will only go on in loyal imitation, I will tell you everything.' The patient did as she was told and was quickly unconscious. When she woke up her canny anaesthetist had gone home.

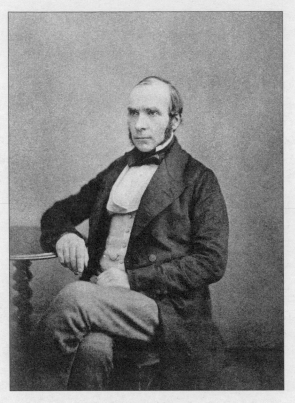

John Snow, aged forty-three

John Snow's growing achievements during the late 1840s and early 1850s changed him hardly at all. The uncompromising, idealistic young man with perhaps a touch of the prig about him, mellowed, as most do, into a more rounded human being, but the modesty, the integrity and the complete lack of acquisitiveness or personal ambition remained. He continued to dress plainly, live simply and to keep to a strict daily routine of work and study, getting up early and retiring to his bed at eleven, in a pattern that was to last to the end of his life.

Most of the hours not taken up by his anaesthesia practice he devoted to research, and by the time of his premature death he had published over eighty books, papers and letters to medical journals on a huge range of subjects, from chest deformities in children to the circulation of the blood, lead poisoning and scarlet fever, and had also given evidence before a Parliamentary committee.

Snow's appearance was as unobtrusive as his personality. He was slim and of medium height, with small features and a calm, gentle expression. The picture that emerges as he moved into middle-age is of a man dedicated to learning and to medicine, whose retiring nature and lack of bedside manner masked a huge compassion. While his reserve made it hard for him to make friends, those who did come to know him, loved him. They discovered loyalty and great kindness, as well as a surprising hidden talent for telling funny anecdotes. 'His long life in comparative student loneliness had made him reserved in manner to strangers; but with private friends he was always open, and of sweet companionship,' Richardson explained. 'With his increased popularity he became less reserved to strangers, and in the last years of his life he so far threw off restraint as to visit the opera occasionally.'

Richardson could never persuade Snow that reading novels was anything other than a frivolous waste of time but said his friend enjoyed the 'ridiculous life pictures' found in the works of some of the most popular writers as much as anyone. 'When he came to see me and leisure was with us, I often read to him some of the more amusing passages from Dickens and Thackeray or Swift. It was a new world to him, and provoked great fun. He would ask to have passages read over again, that he might better realise the conception.'

Richardson sometimes went to even greater lengths in his determination to tease out his friend's lighter side. 'On occasions I would, in ridiculous mood, sing him absurd songs to any tune, two or three tunes, or to no tune at all, and without any pretence at voice,' Richardson recalled. 'At first he would listen with his hands flat together and with a perfect melancholy on his face, as if he could bear it no longer. Bit by bit, he would relax and at last get into a continued laughter. Then I would stop, and he would begin to open out his list of anecdotes, professional and general, upon which the laughter came over to me with compound interest.'

Richardson, who was later knighted for his services to humanitarian causes, had been destined for medicine from the age of ten. His mother on her deathbed had made the young boy promise that he would enter what she told him was the noblest profession in the world, and Richardson never regretted doing so. He first came across John Snow in 1850, when he was twenty-two and Snow was thirty-seven, at the Medical Society of London (formerly the Westminster Medical Society), and the pair were drawn together by their interest in the new speciality of anaesthesia. At a Medical Society meeting in 1853, for example, the *Lancet* reports Richardson reading a paper on 'The Anaesthetic Properties of the Lycoperdon Proteus – the Common Puffball', after which 'Dr Snow corroborated Mr Richardson's observations, having witnessed several of his experiments.' By then, their occasional professional collaboration had developed into a close and lasting friendship.

Richardson later also joined the London Epidemiological Society where Snow was a founder member. This body was set up in 1850 to study epidemic disease and, like the Medical Society of London, held regular meetings where doctors presented papers and discussed the big questions of the day. Other early members included Thomas Addison, who identified pernicious anaemia, as well as the hormonal disorder called Addison's disease, and Richard Bright, a pioneer in the study of kidney disease. At a meeting in 1853 Snow read a paper of his own, comparing the mortality rate in large towns with that in rural districts and discussing some ideas about why urban life was so unhealthy.

Snow's anaesthesia practice had brought him financial security at last, but he was never to earn more than £1,000 a year (about £57,000) – hardly a fortune for a physician attending the rich and famous – largely because he regularly treated poorer patients for no fee. And he also gave some of those earnings away to friends who were struggling, according to Richardson. He was as generous with his time as he was with his money, despite his shyness always giving callers the impression that he had nothing more important to do than to attend to them and was completely at their disposal. When Richardson and Snow first met, Richardson was living at Mortlake, a village on the Thames south-west of London, where his busy practice included looking after several gypsy families. Snow would travel down to help him at the end of his own day's work whenever Richardson asked, often to see a poor, non-paying patient, 'returning as cheerily as though he had received the heaviest fee,' Richardson said, adding: 'All who knew him said he was a quiet man, very reserved and peculiar, a clever man, but not easy to be understood.'

Throughout those years that Snow was experimenting with anaesthesia and building up his practice, however, he had not forgotten one of his much earlier special interests. In 1848 – just as the news of Simpson's discovery broke and as chloroform was being hailed as yet another breakthrough in the long quest to conquer pain – this reserved, clever, 'peculiar' man was confronted once again with another, very different, area of medicine that intrigued him just as much as anaesthesia, and that was now once again crying out for his attention.

Cholera was back.

CHAPTER 7

A Shameful State of Affairs

The case is a lesson in the humanities, the only consolation of which
will be the hope that those poor little victims have not died in vain

Morning Chronicle, January 1849

In the winter of 1848–9, officialdom poked its nose into Mr.
Drouet's Pauper Asylum for Children in the then leafy village of
Tooting, south-west of London. What it found there shocked comfortable Victorian society to its core. Fourteen hundred gaunt-faced
children, some as young as three, were starved half to death, their
bellies swollen, their arms and legs like sticks, their joints deformed
and their skin covered with boils and ulcers. Impetigo and scabies
were endemic, and some of the children bore signs of violence.

Drouet's was one of the infamous child farms where parishes
sent their destitute young charges when their workhouses were
full. Here children who were orphaned or whose parents couldn't
afford to keep them were shut away and largely forgotten, at the
mercy of proprietors who, even if they didn't happen to be sadists
or paedophiles, were in the business to make money. The less spent
on the children's food, clothing and care, the fatter the profits to
be had.

The system had had its critics over the years, and more than a
decade had passed since Charles Dickens described the fate of the

young Oliver Twist at a small farm for very young children. 'The parish authorities magnanimously and humanely resolved that Oliver should be "farmed" or, in other words, that he should be despatched to a branch-workhouse some three miles off, where twenty or thirty other juvenile offenders against the poor-laws rolled about the floor all day, without the inconvenience of too much food or too much clothing, under the parental superintendence of an elderly female who received the culprits at and for the consideration of sevenpence-halfpenny per small head per week,' Dickens wrote. 'The elderly female was a woman of wisdom and experience; she knew what was good for children; and she had a very accurate perception of what was good for herself. So, she appropriated the greater part of the weekly stipend to her own use, and consigned the rising parochial generation to even a shorter allowance than was originally provided for them.'

But despite the efforts of Dickens and other campaigners, it was to take an outbreak of cholera to put a stop to child-farming once and for all. In 1848, after a sixteen-year lull, the still unexplained, untreatable disease was once again advancing upon Britain from India in a second epidemic, largely following the same route it had taken in the 1820s and '30s. That summer, James Yeames, the British consul in Odessa on the Black Sea who had sent warnings to Lord Heytesbury twenty years before, was once more reporting violent outbreaks in his part of the Tsarist empire, and by the end of July, St Petersburg had suffered over 10,000 deaths and Moscow over 9,000.

Again, there was more heat than light about how and why the disease was spreading. Just as in 1831 when Dr Clanny had noted the toads and thunderstorms in Sunderland and wondered what they might portend, Captain Cecil Johnson wrote from Serbia to describe an extraordinary phenomenon. The valley where he lived was overwhelmed by a gigantic swarm of caterpillars that destroyed every plant in their path. The local peasants turned out at dawn with brooms and tree branches to try to beat them back, Johnson said: 'The roads were literally black with them, and the house in which I live was covered to the first floor.' Like Clanny, he also asked if the accompanying strange weather had any significance: 'The heat is overpowering, a breeze blowing like the hot winds of India . . . it is certainly a singular co-incidence that most of the valleys . . . should have been covered with caterpillars of a peculiar kind just as the cholera was advancing to within a few leagues.' Was it only 'a singular co-incidence' or, as Johnson clearly believed, something more?

By August 1848, the disease was again at the Baltic ports, and this time no one was denouncing the stories as scaremongering or suggesting that Britain might be spared. The first official British case was in London in September. John Harnold was a merchant seaman who arrived by the Elbe steamer from Hamburg where cholera was rife. He left his ship and found lodgings by the docks on the south bank of the Thames near Tower Bridge in an area then known as Horsleydown, a small patch of dirty lanes and dilapidated rooming houses. A few days later, Harnold was seized with cholera and within hours he was dead. The following week, a lodger named Blenkinsopp who had taken Harnold's room was also attacked and he too died. Blenkinsopp was only the second case after Harnold in the capital since 1832, which seemed to some to suggest a clear case of contagion.

The government responded in the only way it knew, by setting up another Board of Health. The previous Board had been wound down in December 1832 as the epidemic died away, and, even though for the last few months Sir Henry Halford and his friends had been replaced by a new team more directly under the control of the Privy Council, all of their efforts appeared in vain. This time, then, no doctors held the top jobs. Instead, to the fury of the medical profession, the Board was to be run by a lay trio consisting of Lords Morpeth and Ashley, and Edwin Chadwick. The *Lancet*, never at a loss for a flowery insult, dubbed them 'a benighted triumvirate' who should be ostracised and 'left to the vacillations of their acknowledged ignorance'. The announcement that a close ally of Chadwick's, Thomas Southwood-Smith, MD, had been appointed medical advisor only made matters worse, for the doctor was to be a junior member, lower in status to the others.

Lord Morpeth, the eldest son of Francis Howard, sixth Earl of Carlisle, was a prominent Whig politician. Resigning from a so-called 'pocket borough' parliamentary seat, which was in the gift of his father, Morpeth had gone on to fight and win a seat through an openly contested election and had spent six years as Chief Secretary for Ireland.

Anthony Ashley Cooper, Lord Ashley, is much better known as the Earl of Shaftesbury, a title he was to inherit on the death of his father in 1851. An aristocratic, remote figure who tended to take any criticism of his ideas as a personal insult, he was nevertheless a lifelong campaigner against injustice and cruelty wherever he found it. The name of Shaftesbury is linked with the end of some of the worst excesses of the industrial revolution, which saw young children slaving day and night in the great cotton mills, women and children labouring underground in coal mines and the chimney sweeps' apprentices – the so-called 'climbing boys' – risking serious injury on a daily basis. In the latter campaign, Shaftesbury was helped by Charles Kingsley, the author of *The Water Babies*.

Of the three, however, Edwin Chadwick was by far the most powerful personality. A lawyer-turned-social reformer, admired and loathed in equal measure, six years earlier Chadwick had produced a ground-breaking report into the living and working conditions of the Victorian poor. And in typical forthright Chadwick style, the author had not flinched from detailing exactly what daily life was like for those at the bottom of the heap. In September 1840, for example, Chadwick had personally toured the slums of Glasgow, and one of his team described what they found:

We entered a dirty low passage which led from the street through the first house to a square court, immediately behind which . . . was . . . a dung receptacle of the most disgusting kind. Beyond this court the second passage led to a second court occupied in

the same way by its dunghill; and from this court there was yet
a third passage leading to a third court and a third dungheap.
There were no privies or drains there and the dungheaps received
all the filth which the swarm of wretched inhabitants could give.

The residents, it turned out, paid their rent by selling the contents of the dungheaps as fertiliser.

'The interiors of these houses and their inmates corresponded
with the exteriors,' the inspector continues. 'We saw half-dressed
wretches crowding together to be warm; and in one bed, although
in the middle of the day, several women were imprisoned under a
blanket because as many others who had on their backs all the articles of dress that belonged to the party were then out of doors in
the streets.'

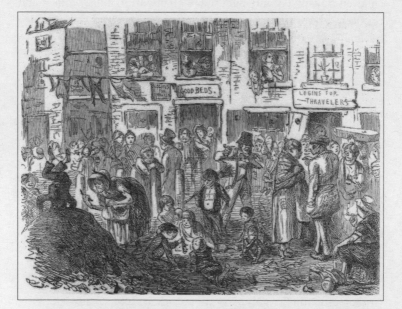

'A court for King Cholera': this 1852 cartoon of the living conditions
of the poor makes the link between dirt and disease

Conditions in the countryside were seldom much better. William Eddy, who worked in a lead mine in Cumberland, told Chadwick about the accommodation provided by his employers:

> Our lodging rooms were such as not to be fit for swine. In one house there were sixteen bedsteads in the room upstairs and fifty occupied these beds at the same time. We could not always get in together but we got in when we could, often three at a time in the bed and one at the foot. I have several times had to get out of bed and sit up all night to make room for my little brothers. There was not a single flag or board on the lower floor and there were pools of water twelve inches deep. You might have taken a coal rake and raked off the dirt and potato peelings six inches deep.

With Edwin Chadwick and his exposés of conditions like these lay the beginnings of our modern concept of public health. An ardent miasmatist – he once announced to a committee of MPs that 'All smell is disease'– Chadwick convinced the nation of the link between filth and illness, and of the need to clean up Britain's towns and cities. In this he was clearly right, albeit for the wrong reasons. In fact, under Chadwick this new board was more a Board of Sanitary Works than a Board of Health, as Lord Morpeth candidly admitted to an incandescent Royal College of Physicians.

Impatient, judgemental and infamously rude, Chadwick, despite his zeal for improving the lot of the working classes, nevertheless believed that the poor were largely to blame for their own misfortunes and, a fierce proponent of what is now called the nanny state, he deemed it the authorities' duty to force people to live prudent, industrious and healthy lives, whether they liked it or not. He also believed in taking power away from the local parishes and putting it firmly into the hands of central government, and he had absolutely no time for what he regarded as irritating nonsense about individual rights. No sooner, then, had Chadwick settled into his Whitehall chair in that autumn of 1848, than with his customary energy and arrogance he began issuing a stream of advice and guidelines. Vegetables, salads and pickles were to be avoided at all costs, the Board announced. Covent Garden came to a standstill and the price of meat shot through the roof. The doctors predicted that any cholera epidemic would soon be eclipsed by a scurvy epidemic. 'Grown-up men and women tremble at a Brussel sprout or a gherkin,' mocked the *Lancet*.

Panic could itself cause the disease, the Board warned but, even so, at the first hint of diarrhoea, people should take twenty grains of candied opium, then readily available, to be repeated every three or four hours, or more often in severe cases. If this piece of amateur prescribing were not irritating enough to medical sensibilities, there was an unfortunate confusion over the recommended dose. The Board had managed to overlook the fact that in England opiate confection consisted of one grain of opium in thirty-six grains of sugar, while in Scotland it was one in forty-three and in Ireland one in twenty-five. The doctors had a field day.

Chadwick had to withdraw much of his advice almost immediately but while making a fool of himself in medical territory, his miasmatism led to some genuinely useful suggestions for public health generally. All public thoroughfares and private alleys and courtyards should be washed down at least once a day, he recommended. Filthy, 'unwholesome' houses or those near bad drains or cesspools should be scrubbed and whitewashed. The parish authorities should inspect and remedy all potential health hazards, such as foul privies and piles of excrement or rubbish. Medical officers should report all cases of epidemic disease. Yet the sad truth was that for all Chadwick's industry, his legal powers were strictly limited: the parishes were free to ignore almost everything he said.

And, of course, as far as the disease about which he was supposed to be guiding the nation was concerned, Chadwick was every inch as ignorant as Sir Henry Halford before him, while the medical profession, for all its glee at the Board's gaffes, remained as confused as ever. When the doctors weren't rowing with Chadwick, they were rowing with each other just as in 1831. All the old remedies – the bizarre, the lethal and the merely useless – were dusted down and fought over once again. And there were some new suggestions.

One medical man, for instance, had heard of naphtha [petrol], being used to good effect by the Russian army in the Caucasus, while surgeon William John Thomas from Liverpool had worked out a treatment plan based on algebraic equations. Rather than use all of the available remedies in one concentrated attack, Thomas argued, doctors should stage their treatments so as to 'oppose power against power to balance the powers of the disease, and to give the powers of the constitution time to rally from the first terrors of the attack'. His long, complicated mathematical formulae for ensuring that the response matched the progress of the disease began: 'Let "d" represent the morbid powers; let "u" represent the force of the remedial powers and let "t" represent the element of time.' Correctly followed, Thomas was sure that his method would prove effective in combating 'the invisible Hannibal from the banks of the Ganges'.

Galvanism, or electric shock treatment, enjoyed some slight popularity for a while, and it was used with seeming success on a little girl of eight who arrived at a London hospital in what appeared to be the last stages of cholera, scarcely breathing, with no pulse at her wrists and a recorded temperature of just 88°F. 'Slight shocks were then passed at short intervals for about a quarter of an hour from the side of the neck to the epigastrium [the area just above the stomach],' her doctor wrote. 'Immediately she opened her eyes and complained of the pain, breathed more fully, pulse became perceptible and temperature rose to 92. Was well in a few days.' As Sir Gilbert Blane had pointed out nearly thirty years earlier, however, by trying out different treatments in this ad hoc, uncontrolled way, doctors ran the risk of congratulating themselves on a cure when there might only have been a happy escape.

Dr Willemin, a Cairo-based physician, had a different idea. He read a scientific paper at a medical conference in Paris in which he claimed to have cured himself of cholera with tincture of cannabis. His theory was that cholera killed by paralysing the nervous system, but that cannabis had a stimulating effect, thus reversing the disease's action. Back in Britain, meanwhile, smoking was under scrutiny. A medical committee decided that convicts on board a prison ship moored at Woolwich docks should be allowed pipes and tobacco after one of their number went down with cholera. Their reasoning was not entirely clear. One London doctor, Richard Horton, was outraged. He said that this would naturally lead the public to think that smoking offered some protection, but, on the contrary, tobacco was a poison that damaged the brain, stomach and heart and caused sickness, headaches, extreme prostration and, in some cases, convulsions, collapse and death.

However, another doctor who gave himself the pseudonym 'A tobacco smoker' took issue with Horton and rushed to defend what he called the soothing weed. Smoking gave excellent protection against cholera, he believed, first 'by relieving the mind from that most depressing agent, fear', and second, by 'neutralising the miasm . . . or . . . disguising noxious effluvia'; in other words, by purifying the air, just as the advocates of chlorine gas and gunpowder had argued. 'I have been a smoker well nigh fifteen years,' he proclaimed, 'and must plead not guilty so far as having been subject to the horrifying symptoms enumerated by Mr Horton . . . In truth, will not every [such] symptom . . . be produced by brandy, and even opium, if improperly administered, yet who would on that account interdict them?

And new ideas about the causes of cholera and its means of spreading, continued apace. One doctor reported that a hugely strong magnet in Moscow had lost its powers when cholera was rife: this should have been investigated. And a fellow theorist wondered if the new railways could be to blame – perhaps the engines and carriages were interfering with the electrical charge in the atmosphere and in some way encouraging the spread of the disease? If so, then beds with glass legs and gutta-percha [natural plastic] shoe-soles might be beneficial, he thought.

Tragically, though, once again all the medical arguments and all the government's advice were for nothing. This epidemic was to prove twice as deadly as the first, and it killed as many as 52,000 people in Britain before it was done. By the spring of 1849, the disease was reported in forty-four towns in England, Scotland and Wales, and in twelve London parishes. 'Cholera is now upon us in full earnest,' wrote Thomas Wakley in the *Lancet* that summer, 'and we verily believe that for all the purposes of protection, three dogs might have been set to bark at the disease with nearly or quite as much efficiency as the paper-braying of Messrs Carlisle [Lord Morpeth], Ashley and Chadwick.'

The disease spread slowly in the capital at first, and in the two months after Harnold and Blenkinsopp died, there were few other recorded cases in London. Then, in December 1848, while Chadwick was starting to pack the pages of the *London Gazette* with recommendations, a virulent outbreak of cholera hit the already badly debilitated children in Mr. Drouet's Pauper Asylum, otherwise known by the misleadingly elegant title of Surrey Hall. In truth, the place was a ramshackle collection of dingy buildings set in low-lying fields under stagnant water.

Three girls had gone down with vomiting and diarrhoea in mid-December, but this was not uncommon, and none of the staff at Drouet's had taken much notice. The first that the authorities heard of a problem was on 1 January, when the father of two of the children told the Holborn Board of Guardians, the parish authority responsible for the poor, that scores of young inmates were desperately ill and dying. When the reports reached Whitehall a few days later, Chadwick dispatched Richard Grainger to investigate. Dr Grainger – a lecturer at St Thomas's Hospital, a fellow of the Royal Society and member of the council of the Royal College of Surgeons – duly set off for Tooting prepared to be confronted with cases of cholera. He arrived on 5 January and went straight to see the sick children.

'I first entered those [rooms] on the female side,' he reported. 'I was struck by a sense of the extreme closeness, oppression and foulness of the air, far exceeding anything I have ever yet witnessed in apartments in hospitals or elsewhere, occupied by the sick . . . The rooms were crowded with beds, utterly disproportionate in number to the space allotted to them. In a room, for example, 16 feet long, 12 feet wide and less than eight feet high, there were five beds occupied by eleven children, all ill with cholera.' In another room, he discovered four girls to a bed. In one room in the boys' section there were eighteen tightly packed beds containing twenty-five very ill children, while ten more boys were sitting around a fire, and one had just died. There were just two nurses trying to look after hundreds of patients. And worse was to come: 'I found that the children were continually vomiting in the beds and on the floor, and that consequently the sheets, bedding and floor were covered with the discharges; and that no efficient aid was in a single case afforded to those suffering children.'

'As a medical man,' Grainger continued, 'it is my duty to state that it is impossible to conceive a state of things more entirely unsuited as to the construction of the buildings and the over-crowding of the inmates, the absence of all efficient nursing and the want of the recognised means of medical and other treatment, than was presented in this establishment.'

Grainger then decided to take a stroll around the rest of the premises, and was equally disturbed by what he saw of the children's usual living conditions. The other dormitories and the schoolrooms were dark, airless and full to bursting point. The playground was damp and far too small for the numbers of children; the grounds and surrounding fields were criss-crossed with streams and ditches that stank of excrement, and one building that housed 150 children was next to a yard where large numbers of pigs, cows, horses and poultry were kept in the most appalling squalor. And from what the doctor could see, the children's food, clothing and bedding were totally inadequate.

When Grainger reported back to Whitehall later that afternoon, Chadwick, who could never be accused of procrastination, at once told the London Boards of Guardians to take their children out of Drouet's. Not all of them complied, but most did, and over the next few days hundreds of children were removed to hospital or to the workhouse. Even so, by the end of January, 180 of them had died.

Not surprisingly, once the children had been removed and the immediate emergency was over, questions began to be asked about what, exactly, had been going on at Tooting. The coroner for Surrey, into whose jurisdiction some of the deaths fell, said he saw no reason to hold inquests, but his counterpart for Middlesex disagreed. This was none other than the irascible Thomas Wakley, a doctor and Member of Parliament, who also happened to occupy the editor's chair at the *Lancet* where he spent much of his time goading the likes of Sir Henry Halford, Edwin Chadwick and anyone else whose self-importance he found irritating. The horror stories that began to emerge about Mr Drouet once the indefatigable Wakley took up the case threw Grainger's revelations into the shade.

It appeared, for example, that a Mr Wynch from the Holborn Guardians had gone with two others to inspect the asylum the previous May. They had arrived, he said, to find the boys at dinner. 'They were all standing. I believe they never sit at meals. I cut up 100 potatoes, not one of which was fit to eat . . . They were positively black and diseased . . . I spoke to Mr Drouet, and he said he gave £7 a ton for them. I told him I thought the diet should be changed, and he said if we paid him better he would do it.'

Wynch then asked the boys to put up their hands if they had any complaints about the food. 'About 40 did so. I selected one boy who seemed intelligent for questions. Drouet became very violent and said we were using him unfairly and in an ungentlemanly manner. He called the boys liars and scoundrels and said the one I had selected was the worst in the school . . . said we ought to be satisfied with his word.' Laughter rippled around the courtroom at this last remark.

Sixteen-year-old Thomas Titan, whose task it was to slop out the tubs used as lavatories and to scrub the dormitory floors, then related what had happened once Mr Wynch and his colleagues were safely off the premises. 'After the gentlemen came to ask about our treatment, I heard Mr Drouet say to one of the boys: "I'll let you know, you young scoundrel, for letting them know you had not enough to eat."' The lad was thrashed the following day.

Soon after Grainger returned from his harrowing visit to Tooting, Keziah Dermond, deputy-matron of the Holborn Workhouse, made her way over to London's Royal Free Hospital to prepare for the arrival of 157 sick children whom the Holborn Guardians, on Chadwick's advice, were removing from Drouet's that night. When the first of the young patients began arriving in a fleet of horse-drawn vans, Mrs Dermond, like Grainger, was shocked by what she saw: 'The children were generally very sore in their bodies [that is, covered with sores]. Their feet were in a dreadful state. They were sore and had not been dressed, and there were wounds on different parts of their bodies,' she said. Mary Harris, a nurse at the Royal Free, was detailed to look after six-year-old James Andrews who, too weak to sit up, had made the journey from Tooting on the lap of one of the older boys. 'I gave him some bread and milk, and he said, "Oh nurse, what a big piece of bread this is." He drank the milk but could only eat a portion of the bread,' she explained. 'He appeared very fatigued, and I put him to bed and I observed as I undressed him that he was very thin and emaciated.' James died the next day.

John Woodhouse was luckier. Older and tougher than little James Andrews, he managed to survive his time at Tooting and was eventually able to tell his story. Woodhouse had been sent to Drouet's by the St Pancras Board of Guardians, who were clearly as ineffectual as their Holborn counterparts when it came to the welfare of the children for whom they were responsible: 'When the gentlemen came down, I was afraid to tell them I had not enough to eat, lest the schoolmaster should hear me and beat me,' Woodhouse said. 'Some of the Chelsea boys were beaten for telling the gentlemen of the Chelsea Board they had not enough to eat.' And he added, as though he felt it important that the individuals concerned be known and recorded: 'Those boys names are Rowe and Cutler, but Cutler is now dead.' And Rowe and Cutler had clearly suffered in vain for daring to speak out to the Chelsea Board, for the food at Drouet's had stayed as bad as ever.

Woodhouse then told Wakley what he had been too scared to

tell the St Pancras visitors: 'We always had gruel for breakfast, and I think it was made from flour and water' ("No better than bill-sticker's paste", commented the coroner). 'I never had bread and milk there . . . I have known boys so hungry they have got over the palings to eat the stuff out of the pig tubs.' Woodhouse also described how he and some of the other boys were sent out to work in a local farmer's fields but had received no wages. Presumably Mr Drouet appropriated their money. Woodhouse went on: 'The boys sometimes slept three in a bed, and when they wet the bed, they were put four in a bed as a punishment and had to lie on cold oil-cloth.'

The girls fared no better. One nine-year-old was carried into court in the arms of a nurse, wrapped in a blanket like a baby. When Wakley asked if there was anything the matter with her, he was told that she was very ill with scabies. 'On the blanket being opened, the lower part of the legs were found to be covered with rags, but sufficient of the feet and legs were visible to show that the flesh was covered with brown marks, which were said to extend in the same manner all over the body of the unfortunate girl,' wrote a reporter from the *Morning Chronicle*. Mr Goodrich, the medical attendant of the Hanover Square Workhouse in central London, then told the court that in all his thirty years' experience he had never seen such a dreadful case.

One of the St Pancras girls called Jane Alford told Wakley: 'We had not enough bread to eat, nor anything else . . . We were not warm enough . . . I was afraid to complain because the girls said if I did, Miss Day, the matron, would box my ears. When we washed we had no soap nor towels, and had to wipe ourselves on our pinafores.' Some of the girls also had more than neglect and blows to contend with. The Kensington Guardians, to their credit, had removed their girls from Drouet's in November, 'in consequence of the complaints of some of them that Mr Drouet's brother had acted improperly towards them'.

And so it went on. Day after day, a seemingly never-ending procession of doctors, nurses, workhouse officials, members of Boards of

Guardians, bereaved parents and surviving children trooped into court to give their shaming testimonies. And if any more help were needed in whipping up public indignation, Wakley and Grainger found that they had the most powerful of allies. The signature on Dr Grainger's report was that of the secretary to Chadwick's Board, one Henry Austin, an architect and engineer by training who had once helped Robert Stephenson to build a railway line. Austin's shock at the state of the slums through which the track was to pass had led him to become an active campaigner for better housing for the poor and thus a friend of Chadwick, and it so happened that Austin had a family connection that ensured the message of Tooting was spelt out in no uncertain terms to the nation. Austin's wife, Laetitia, was the sister of Charles Dickens.

On 20 January 1849, the front page of the weekly newspaper, the *Examiner*, carried an unsigned article under the heading, 'The Paradise at Tooting'. The author began by lampooning the panic-stricken attempts of some of the Guardians when news of the epidemic first broke to paint a benign picture of Mr Drouet, and therefore clear themselves from any blame.

'Of all similar establishments on earth, that at Tooting was the most admirable,' the piece ran.

Of all similar contractors on earth, Mr Drouet was the most disinterested, zealous and unimpeachable. Of all the wonders ever wondered at, nothing perhaps had ever occurred more wonderful than the outbreak and rapid increase of a disorder so horrible, in a place so perfectly regulated. There was no warning of its approach. Nothing was less to be expected. The farmed children were slumbering in the lap of peace and plenty; Mr Drouet, the farmer, was slumbering with an easy conscience, but with one eye perpetually open, to keep watch upon the blessings he diffused, and upon the happy infants under his paternal charge; when, in a moment, the destroyer was upon them, and Tooting church-yard became too small for the piles of children's coffins that were carried out of this Elysium every day.

Then, after a side-swipe at the Surrey coroner who had deemed it unnecessary to inquire into the deaths, the writer goes on to praise Wakley who, he says, 'being of little faith, holds inquests, and even manifests a disposition to institute a very searching inquiry into the causes of these horrors; rather thinking that such grievous effects must have some grievous cause . . .'

> It then comes out – the truth is so perverse – that Mr Drouet is not altogether that golden farmer he was supposed to be . . . He has a bad habit of putting four cholera patients in one bed. He has a weakness in respect of leaving the sick to take care of themselves, surrounded by every offensive, indecent and barbarous circumstance that can aggravate the horrors of their condition and increase the dangers of infection . . . His establishment is crammed . . . The diet of the children is so unwholesome and insufficient that they climb secretly over palings and pick out scraps of sustenance from the tubs of hog-wash. Their clothing by day and their covering by night are shamefully defective. Their rooms are cold, damp, dirty and rotten. In a word, the age of miracles is past, and of all conceivable places in which pestilence might – or rather must – be expected to break out and to make direful ravages, Mr Drouet's model farm stands foremost.

The anonymous author of this elegant and powerful piece of polemic was, of course, Charles Dickens.

The day after his visit to Drouet's, Dr Grainger delivered a lecture to a huge audience in the great hall of St Thomas's Hospital in London, in which he made plain his belief that cholera, which he held to be a disease of the blood, was not contagious. If it were, then nothing would be able to stop it, he argued, and in a classic piece of miasmatism, he reminded his listeners that those of the Hamburg poor who lived near stagnant ditches had been hit five times harder than the poor in other parts of the city; and that Glasgow – where filth and overcrowding were beyond imagining, he said – had had as many as 140 cases a day. Two weeks later, Grainger was appearing before a different public, as a witness at the inquest into the death of James Andrews. He described how he and a colleague had examined 560 pale sickly Drouet children, with their weak limbs and distended bellies, and gave it as his opinion that: 'The children were predisposed to the attack [of cholera] by insufficient food, insufficient clothing, and the noxious influences of an atmosphere arising from the stagnant ditches and putrid water of the neighbourhood.'

Chadwick, with his interest in the link between health and the environment, had already commissioned a surveyor's report of Drouet's land and buildings. This revealed that the fields around the asylum were being used as dumping grounds for the sewage of Tooting, and, not surprisingly, that the ditches were full of 'filthy deposits, emitting offensive emanations'. When the wind was in a certain quarter, the report concluded, 'The foul emanations . . . would be wafted towards Mr Drouet's establishment, and must exercise a prejudicial effect on the health of the inmates.'

On 23 January, the coroner's jury at the Holborn inquest announced its verdict: Bartholomew Peter Drouet was guilty of manslaughter. The jury then went on to attack the Holborn Guardians, who had acted 'most negligently in their engagement with Mr Drouet and also with regard to their visits to his establishment'. However, one person was singled out for exemption from blame. Mr Wynch, who had tackled Drouet over the potatoes, 'had done his duty, so far as lay in his power,' the jury found. When the verdict came in, Drouet had long since gone home, and so Wakley issued a warrant for his arrest.

The criminal trial opened at London's famous Central Criminal Court on 13 April 1849. Drouet stood in the Old Bailey dock charged first with the manslaughter of James Andrews 'by omitting to provide him with proper food, nourishment, sleeping accommodation and clothing to protect him from the inclemency of the weather', and then, similarly, with the manslaughter of four other Holborn children. He pleaded not guilty to all charges. After little

more than a day of harrowing evidence, the case suddenly collapsed. Mr Justice Platt stopped the proceedings and ordered the
jury to return a 'Not guilty' verdict on the grounds that they had
heard nothing to show that little James Andrews would have survived the attack of cholera that killed him, had he never been so
unfortunate as to fall into the hands of Mr Drouet.

Most commentators agreed that the prosecution case had been
badly handled, but the underlying problem with obtaining a conviction, despite all that had come out at the inquests and the
subsequent trial, was that no one knew enough about cholera to be
certain how much Drouet's treatment, appalling though it unques-
tionably was, had contributed to the boy's death. Witness after
witness had testified to the fact that Drouet had omitted to provide
James Andrews with 'proper food, nourishment, sleeping accommodation and clothing', but was this why the child had died?
Would he have withstood the disease if he had been well nourished
and properly clothed? And did the cholera only strike at Drouet's
in the first place because of the filth and overcrowding? Was
Dickens right when he asserted: 'Of all conceivable places in which
pestilence might – or rather must – be expected to break out and to
make direful ravages, Mr Drouet's model farm stands foremost'?
Was Grainger right in blaming a lack of food and warm clothing
combined with the stink from the putrid ditches of Tooting? No
one really knew.

Drouet left the dock in tears. 'It might be gratitude for his escape
or it might be grief that his occupation was put an end to,' commented the *Examiner*, clearly considering remorse an unlikely
explanation for this show of emotion. But while the man most
people considered personally responsible for the deaths of 180
children was being allowed to walk free, there was one satisfactory outcome from the affair. Thomas Wakley, who described Mr
Justice Platt's decision as 'tantamount to a judicial declaration that
death by Asiatic cholera was death by the visitation of God, altogether irrespective of starvation and overcrowding', believed that
a great result had, nevertheless, been obtained. 'Child farming, like

military flogging, is virtually abolished,' he declared, and he was right. Legislation was unnecessary. Thanks to Mr Drouet, no parish in the country would now dare send its young dependants to such places.

John Snow could only watch as the tragedy was played out that winter. At the time, he was busily building up his anaesthesia practice. He had published his classic textbook, *On the Inhalation of the Vapour Ether in Surgical Operations*, the previous year, and by 1848 was switching his attention to James Simpson's latest discovery, chloroform. During all the years that had passed since his time at Killingworth Colliery, however, while he completed his training at the Westminster and set himself up as a medical man in the capital, he had continued to ponder the cholera mystery, and some ideas had taken root in his mind. Now as the details emerged from the scandal at Tooting, he saw more evidence to support his growing theory and to convince him that he was, at last, closing in on the answer.

As with those terrible days at Killingworth, Snow, for all his compassion and his personal kindness, was able to look beyond the immediate horror of Drouet's to concentrate on what actually happened when cholera struck. Again, he thought about the disease's initial symptoms and its action upon the body. And again he thought about how the 'poison' appeared to spread. He was also intrigued by some striking similarities between the living conditions at Drouet's and the working conditions in coal mines. His brother Robert was a pit manager at a colliery near Leeds and knew all the unsavoury details: 'Our colliers descend at five o'clock in the morning, to be ready for work at six, and leave the pit from one to half-past three,' he told John. 'The average time spent in the pit is eight to nine hours. The pitmen all take down with them a supply of food ... I fear that our colliers are no better than others as regards cleanliness. The pit is one huge privy, and of course the men always take their victuals with unwashed hands.'

Snow compared this with what Grainger had found at Tooting. Here the children were crammed two, three or even four to a bed, the cholera victims often mixed in with healthy children and left, uncared for, to vomit over everything and everyone. He also thought about how children get their hands into everything and are always putting their fingers in their mouths. He thought about the unfortunate Harnold and Blenkinsopp and their squalid room at Horsleydown – and he was very interested indeed to hear about an unremarkable London street called Albion Terrace in Battersea, just over the river from Chelsea.

CHAPTER 8

A Little Light

The belief in the communication [person-to-person transmission] of cholera is a much less dreary one than the reverse; for what is so dismal as the idea of some invisible agent pervading the atmosphere and spreading over the world?

John Snow, 1849

Albion Terrace, Battersea, was a neat row of genteel suburban dwellings inhabited by the professional classes and the better-off tradesmen, a world away from the lodging houses of Horsleydown or the dormitories of Drouet's asylum. Here clean, well-nourished people – stockbrokers, lawyers, doctors, the backbone of society – lived comfortable, orderly lives. No one dossed down in a grimy bed, still warm from another man's body, or supplemented their diet from the pig-swill bin.

Yet during two weeks in the summer of 1849, nine months after Harnold and Blenkinsopp died and three months after Bartholomew Drouet left the dock at the Old Bailey without a legal stain on his character, more than half of the residents of ten of the seventeen houses in the street went down with cholera, and twenty-four of them died. Among the victims was a household of six people, including one who fled London in an attempt to escape both the scene of his grief and the cholera. Meanwhile, all of the surrounding streets stayed entirely free from disease.

The drama began on 28 July. A middle-aged servant at number 13 had had sickness and diarrhoea for a few days; her illness was unpleasant, as sickness and diarrhoea always are, but appeared to be the result of no more than a routine stomach upset. The warning bells rang when she collapsed suddenly and died within hours. Two days later her sister, who had come up from the country to look after her, also dropped dead with no warning. And so it continued. One after the other for the next ten days, the respectable residents of Albion Terrace fell sick and died of Asiatic cholera.

The worst tragedy was played out at number 6, where the Reverend Thomas Harrison, a sixty-one-year-old retired missionary, lived with his wife and an elderly cook. At the time, Harrison's aunt, Mrs Roscoe, and her friend Mrs Edwards were on a visit to Battersea, after which they all planned a trip to Brighton. Instead, on Saturday 4 August, Henrietta Roscoe died of cholera, leaving her considerable fortune to the clergyman. He was not to enjoy it. On the following Tuesday Martha Edwards, Ann Harrison and a nurse called Mary Blackwell who had been hired to look after them, all died. Two days after that, Mrs Edward's nephew, a young man called Jenkins, stood and watched at Kensal Green cemetery, the sole mourner as the three women were buried in the same grave into which Mrs Roscoe had only just been laid to rest. When Jenkins returned to Albion Terrace, he discovered that a second nurse had died in the short time that he was at the funeral.

As Mrs Harrison and Mrs Edwards lay dying that Tuesday evening, Thomas Harrison had had a visit from his next-door neighbour, a lawyer called Maxwell. Mr Maxwell sat up all night with the distraught man, and at six o'clock the next morning, with his wife and aunt now dead in their beds, Harrison told his friend that he couldn't bear to stay in the house a moment longer and would never set foot in the place again. Maxwell ran out into the quiet suburban streets in search of a hackney carriage, and the pair then set off at speed in the early summer light for Jack Straw's Castle, a famous old inn in the rural eighteenth-century village of

Hampstead, to the north-west of London. They had no sooner arrived, however, when the minister began to feel ominously sick and, realising what must inevitably lie in store for him, he asked the lawyer to do him one last favour – to write out his will, disposing of the money that Mrs Roscoe had left him just three days before. Eight hours later the Reverend Thomas Harrison was dead. He had seen his relatives and servants die before him and, said *The Times*, 'could not fly from the poison which he carried in his breast'. The sole survivor at number 6 Albion Terrace was an ageing cook.

By 1849, stories of this kind were only too commonplace in the tenements, the cottages and the great workhouses and prisons, but such an attack on the affluent middle classes was extraordinary, and it brought with it the evidence that John Snow had been waiting for. The previous autumn, as Britain's second epidemic began to take hold, the ideas that Snow had long been pondering about cholera's method of attack and means of transmission began to come together in his mind to form a coherent theory.

He outlined his thinking to a few other doctors with an interest in the subject, notably Edmund Parkes and Alfred Baring Garrod of University College Hospital, who were busily analysing the blood and discharges of large numbers of cholera patients in what was proving a vain hope of finding something, anything, that might shed some light on the mystery. Parkes – like Daun and Russell who had played such key roles in 1831 – had been an army doctor in India, where he had seen up close diseases such as dysentery, hepatitis and cholera, and he would go on to make his name in the newly developing field known as medical hygiene. Parkes was not impressed by Snow's theory. In his view, Snow was placing far more weight on one particular idea than was justified by the then known facts and, looking back some years later, Parkes would blame what he saw as Snow's exclusivity of thinking for the prejudice shown against his theory. It was no wonder that Snow's ideas gained little credence when he dismissed some other strong contenders long before they had been disproved, Parkes believed.

That autumn, Snow had agreed with Parkes insofar as he thought the information he had collected to date was too flimsy to justify the publication of an academic paper. But now as the story of Albion Terrace began to emerge, he found that he had some facts within his grasp, if not to prove his case beyond doubt, then certainly to allow him to put forward a credible argument. 'The opinions now made known have been entertained by the author since the latter part of last year and were mentioned by him to several medical gentlemen,' he wrote, 'but he hesitated to publish them, thinking the evidence in their favour so scattered and general as not to be likely to make a ready and easy impression. Within the last few days, however, some occurrences have come within his knowledge which seem to offer more direct proof.'

As soon as news of the events at Battersea came to Edwin Chadwick's ear, he ordered another of his inquiries, and one of Dr Grainger's colleagues, a Dr Milroy, duly wrote a report on the affair, singling out three factors for blame: first, the bad smell from an open sewer in a piece of land known as Battersea Fields some 400 feet away from the houses; second, bad smells from the kitchen sinks in Albion Terrace, which had become much worse after a drain burst in a storm just two days before the first victim died, flooding two of the houses; and lastly, the smell from a huge pile of rubbish, equivalent to eight cart-loads and swarming with maggots, that had been festering quietly for months in the cellar at number 13, the very house where the first victim died.

In fact, according to Milroy, Albion Terrace was: 'a striking example of the potent agency of foul and putrid effluvia in attracting and localising the malarious poison that is abroad in the atmosphere, causing it to settle down upon the unfortunate residents with the most fatal severity, even when other causes of insalubrity are absent'. Put more simply, at a time when cholera was rife in the air, the smells at Albion Terrace had been so strong that they alone were enough to cause the outbreak, without any help from other factors such as the malnourishment and over-crowding that were thought to have played a role at Tooting.

Milroy's was an orthodox view in tune with the thinking of most of the medical profession at the time. And it seemed especially convincing given that the first victim lived in the house with the rubbish heap and died just after the basements had flooded, with all the resulting filth and smell. John Snow, however, remained unimpressed: 'With respect to the open sewer, there are several streets and lines of houses as much exposed to any emanations there might be from it as those in which the cholera prevailed; and yet they were quite free from the malady, as were nineteen houses situated between the sewer and Albion Terrace.'

And as for stinking sinks, Snow went on, these were such an everyday feature in practically every kitchen in the land that they could not possibly be responsible for this explosion of disease. In fact, that same rainstorm had caused disgusting smells in thousands of homes right across London; and the inhabitants of the two Albion Terrace houses that had been flooded – and where the smells had consequently been worst – had come off comparatively lightly. His dismissal of Milroy's third culprit, the nasty secret in the cellar at number 13, was, for Snow, almost contemptuous. A smell beneath one house could not possibly have affected houses some distance away, was his only comment.

From Snow's extensive work with anaesthetics and from the incident with arsenic at the Hunterian School all those years before, he knew only too well the dangers of breathing certain chemical vapours and gases, but he did not believe that a mere bad smell in itself could cause a particular epidemic disease. Diseases such as smallpox, scarlet fever and cholera, which had specific symptoms, had to be caused by a specific 'poison', he argued, which developed within the body, whose behaviour was governed by fixed natural laws, and which was passed on from one individual to another. Benjamin Ward Richardson said that Snow believed it was no more illogical to expect a foul smell to cause oak trees to grow in a field or crocuses in a garden than to think that it could cause a particular disease: 'The smallpox may occur over a cesspool, as an oak may spring up through a manure heap, but the smallpox would never appear over the cesspool in the absence of its specific poison, nor the oak rise from the manure heap in the absence of the acorn which seeded it.' Richardson described this as an extreme view, coming as it did when only the first faint glimmerings of a link between micro-organisms and disease were being identified, and some ten years before Louis Pasteur demonstrated beyond doubt the role that germs had to play.

Snow found the work of Mr Grant, the assistant surveyor to the Commissioners of Sewers, far more persuasive than the theories of Dr Milroy. Grant had had the ground behind houses numbers 1 and 7 opened up, and the drains examined. And what the surveyor discovered there persuaded the cautious John Snow into print. Not only did he now have enough information to justify setting out his ideas before a wide audience, he felt, but he had a positive duty to do so in the interests of saving lives.

Albion Terrace received its water supply from a spring in the road that ran along the front of the houses. What was known as a 'barrel' drain ran between the houses at numbers 7 and 8, carrying the water from the spring to the back of the row of houses, from where it was piped to the right and to the left in order to feed the tanks that lay in the ground behind each house. These tanks were connected to each other by a series of pipes, and more pipes then carried the water from each tank to a pump in the kitchens. Behind each house was a cesspool underneath a privy, four feet away from the water tank.

When Grant's men dug down behind the houses at numbers 1 and 7, they found that the cesspools at both houses were full and that the overflow drain at number 1 was blocked. This drain was just fifteen inches above the water tank, the ground between drain and tank was soaking wet, and the bottom of the drain so crumbling and porous that one of the men was able to poke a stick through it. This drain also passed over the pipe that supplied the water tanks, the joints of which were not properly sealed.

Behind number 7, Grant found that the contents of a pipe bringing surplus water from the tanks and the contents of the drain from the cesspool were running into each other. He also uncovered a flat brick drain laid over the top of the barrel drain that brought the water from the spring. Into this flat drain flowed surplus water from the road, waste from the cesspools and the kitchen sinks, and surplus water from the tanks, and it was this drain that had burst during the storm, flooding two houses with effluent. After this, most of the residents had remarked on the bad state of the drinking water. The drain at number 8 also overflowed during more heavy rain at the beginning of August, again flooding two kitchens.

In other words, the contents of the cesspools and the sewers could find their way into the pipes and tanks that supplied the drinking water at Albion Terrace by several different routes and, because the tanks were on the same level and interconnected, anyone pumping water in one kitchen would draw water from the other tanks as well as from their own, causing an impurity in one tank to pollute all the rest.

Grant also took samples of water from the tanks. These, he said, 'required but to be looked at and smelled to satisfy anyone of their contamination, which seems clearly to have taken place after the water left the spring'. Snow was able to get hold of some of these samples for a closer examination, and his description of what he found makes for deeply unpleasant reading: 'The large bottle, labelled no. 7, contains black, semi-fluid matter, possessing very distinctly the odour of privy soil. On proceeding to open the bottle, as soon as the cork was disturbed, it was driven violently out, together with part of the contents, by the gases resulting from the putrification going on.'

And that was not the worst of it: 'Several substances that escape digestion were found in the contents of this bottle – such as currants, grape-stones and portions of the epidermis, or thin outer covering, of fruits and vegetables – and another material that enters privies was found, namely little bits of paper.' As to how it was possible for people to drink such water before realising that it was foul, Snow pointed out that the thicker, more obviously nasty ingredients would sink to the bottom of the tanks, leaving the water that was pumped off looking relatively harmless.

Only four other houses, just around the corner in Albion Street, received the same water as Albion Terrace, but three of these had stood empty for months, and the fourth was occupied by a man who had always suspected the water and never drank it. Thomas Harrison had complained a lot about the taste of the water that summer, and on the day that Mrs Harrison and Mrs Edwards died, he told the cook to throw the tea away and get some more water from the other side of the main road. The cook, the only survivor at number 6, said that she herself had 'grumbled and growled' about the water, and refused to drink it.

In August 1849, then, Snow published a pamphlet explaining his carefully argued hypothesis. First, he reasoned, cholera was clearly contagious – that is, able to be passed on by a sick person to a healthy one. It always followed the main travel routes and, time after time, it would strike a place previously free from disease soon after the arrival of someone from an affected area. Second, whatever caused the disease – the cholera 'poison' – must be entering the body through the alimentary canal; in other words, it had to be swallowed. This was clear from its mode of action, for those terrible, now only too-familiar first symptoms – the violent vomiting and diarrhoea – affected the digestive system alone. Unlike diseases that had their origins in the bloodstream, cholera did not start with general symptoms such as rigor, headache or a fast pulse: its initial action was very local.

The idea that cholera was a blood disorder had come about partly because of the thick, black tar-like substance that passed for blood in the victims' veins and arteries. This must mean that the cholera 'poison' was active in the bloodstream, it was thought, somehow causing the blood's normal water and salt content to pass out of the body through the walls of the stomach and intestines. But Snow argued that this idea ran contrary to everything shown by medical experience. He could think of no other single example in which a poison in the blood caused fluids to be lost through a single surface of the body – in this case, the alimentary canal. Far more likely, he believed, that the fluid loss was due to a local irritation within the digestive system itself.

Working on the theory, then, that cholera was a disorder of the digestive system and not of the blood, the obvious way for a healthy person to catch the disease from a sick person was by swallowing some of the matter thrown off during the illness: the vomit or the massive cloudy discharges – rice-water evacuations – from the bowels. These were often colourless and odourless; traces could get unnoticed on to the hands and then into the mouth of someone nursing a patient. If that person was also preparing meals for a family or handling food for sale then the 'poison' would be spread further, even over quite a distance. This was clearly much more likely to happen among the poor, living in such unhygienic conditions.

What this did not explain, however, was cholera's frightening habit of exploding without warning into a huge epidemic, striking scores or even hundreds of people at the same time. But there was another way that it could spread, a way that it could strike simultaneously on a massive scale, and that was if infected sewage were able to find its way into the water supply. And in the first half of the nineteenth century, this was not only possible, it was almost inevitable, as Mr Grant's investigations at Albion Terrace had demonstrated only too well.

On Albion Terrace, Snow commented: 'It remains evident that the only special and peculiar cause connected with the great calamity which befell the inhabitants of these houses was the state of the water, which was followed by the cholera in almost every house to which it extended, whilst all the surrounding houses were quite free from the disease.' There was a seeming anomaly in the case of two nurses who had caught cholera even though they had only come to Albion Terrace after the outbreak had begun and after the residents had decided that the water was unfit for drinking, but Snow believed that they had contracted the disease either by unknowingly swallowing a trace of vomit or excreta from one of their patients, as he outlined in his pamphlet, or by eating food that had previously been in contact with the tainted water.

No one, John Snow included, had any idea how the servant at number 13 had contracted the disease that sparked off the tragedy in the first place – the index case – any more than anyone knew how cholera had first been introduced into Drouet's asylum. The woman herself was dead, and there was absolutely no information to be had about how she might have been exposed. But Snow believed that he had identified the cause of the other deaths at Albion Terrace: 'There are no data for showing how the disease was communicated to the first patient on 28 July; but it was two or three days afterwards, when the evacuations from this patient must have entered the drains having a communication with the water supplied to all the houses, that other persons were attacked, and in two days more the disease prevailed to an alarming extent,' he wrote.

This was not the first time that anyone had suggested that drinking foul water – as opposed to breathing the bad smell that it gave off – might have a part to play in the spread of cholera. During both the 1831–2 epidemic and this one, investigators had noticed that people had sometimes complained about the foul taste of the water just before falling sick, as the Reverend Thomas Harrison and his neighbours had done. Even Chadwick's Board of Health, that hotbed of miasmatism, acknowledged that when a local water supply was polluted by a sewer or privy or by rainwater seeping in from a nearby graveyard, then any subsequent attacks of cholera proved especially deadly. And Richard Grainger admitted that sometimes it was difficult to arrive at any other conclusion 'than that the use of water polluted by decomposed organic matter acted intensely as a predisposing cause'.

Again, though, here was Grainger seeing contaminated drinking water as just one factor that might make people more susceptible to cholera, not as the primary cause of the disease. He, like Chadwick and Milroy and their many fellow travellers, came at the problem from the absolute conviction that bad smells lay at the root of all epidemic disease. To them, miasmatism was a proven scientific fact rather than a theory based on purely circumstantial evidence, albeit a huge amount of such evidence dating back hundreds of years.

John Snow, by proposing his particular route out of the impasse in which mainstream thinking about the spread of disease now found itself, was also offering the tantalising possibility of a simple, cheap yet hugely effective strategy for stopping cholera in its tracks. For if he were right, then this killer that even now had entire nations in terror, would prove, after all, extraordinarily easy to tame. All that was needed, Snow reasoned, was for everyone looking after a cholera patient to wash their hands thoroughly and often, particularly before touching food, and for people to avoid drinking or cooking with water into which drains and sewers were emptied. And if the latter should prove impossible, then the water should be filtered and boiled before use.

So here it was at last: a brilliant piece of logical deduction, explaining all of cholera's maddening contradictions that had teased the greatest medical brains for so long and with such terrible consequences. At this stage it was, of course, only a theory, albeit a very promising one. Snow had made assumptions and he knew that he needed hard scientific evidence, ideally from conducting some sort of experiment, although it was difficult to see how this could be done. Unlike his work on anaesthetics or arsenic, this theory did not lend itself to laboratory tests. At the very least he would have liked time to collect more data before going into print but with the country in the grip of an epidemic, he thought it indefensible to sit on information that might save lives. So, apologising for what he was the first to point out were the shortcomings of his work, he explained his thinking in a small pamphlet and invited his colleagues to give him their views.

He was to be disappointed. Despite Britain's desperate, corpse-littered search for answers for nearly twenty years, despite the millions who had died across the world in the thirty years since the pandemics began, the medical establishment greeted Snow's work with a resounding silence, just as the members of the Westminster Medical Society had received his first contributions to their debates. No one, it seemed, was much interested in the ideas of an unclubable loner without money or influence who spent every spare hour closeted away with his books and experiments, especially when those ideas ran so contrary to orthodox medical opinion.

A month after Snow's publication appeared, the *Lancet* printed a short review. The writer described Snow's argument that cholera was not a blood disease being spread via the lungs through inhalation, but a local disease of the gut, spread via the digestive system, as 'not by any means decisive'. And his theory about the role of contaminated water should be received 'with great limitation', the journal warned, but it did add that it would be unfair to attempt a precis of Snow's arguments and recommended that medical men read the pamphlet for themselves. There was, however, no suggestion that Snow's advice about disease prevention – advice that practically every person in the country could understand and follow – was at least worth trying at a time when over a thousand lives a week were being lost in Britain alone. And, unusually, no readers reached for their pens to support or denounce him. John Snow didn't even merit howls of derision. They simply ignored him.

CHAPTER 9

Sensation

> In all falling rain, carried from gutters into water-butts, animalcules
> are to be found; and in all kinds of water, standing in the open air,
> animalcules can turn up
>
> Dutch microscopist Antony van Leeuwenhoek, 1702

To the London elite of the medical profession, the microscopical sub-committee of the Bristol Medico-Chirugical [surgical] Society might not have been the most obvious setting for a great scientific discovery but, given the ignorance and confusion about cholera, it was as good as anywhere.

On 9 July 1849, six weeks before John Snow published his ideas, two doctors unveiled some extraordinary findings before their colleagues, gathered at the house of William Budd. Budd, a Devon man from a large medical family and a physician at the Bristol Infirmary, was later to claim his place in medical history with his work on typhoid, distinguishing it once and for all from typhus fever.

Joseph Griffiths Swayne, a lecturer at the Bristol Medical School, and a local surgeon called Frederick Brittan, had taken some samples of the so-called 'rice-water evacuations' from patients in the local cholera hospital and studied them under the microscope. The pair then made drawings of what they found: 'Cells of a very pecu-

liar character which have been hitherto undescribed,' Swayne said.
These bodies were 'in considerable abundance and so singular in
appearance that we expressed our opinion that they were characteristic of the evacuations of cholera, if not the very agents causing
the disease.'

To make sure, they subjected the discharges of another fifty
patients to the same scrutiny. The results were identical. There, as
plain as could be in the fluid under the glass, were particles of a
type that they had never seen before.

Further discoveries came thick and fast. Investigating the air in
a house where five cholera patients were being nursed, Brittan
reported exactly the same strange bodies, while Budd detected
huge numbers in the water supply of the 'cholera' districts. Brittan
and Swayne then compared the cholera evacuations to samples
from people suffering from what the doctors were certain was
simple, non-choleraic diarrhoea, and Budd looked at specimens of
water from districts not affected by the epidemic. None of them
could detect any trace of the weird little bodies. This, they were
sure, was the clincher: they had made a major breakthrough
and were probably looking at the very poison that caused
cholera.

On 29 September 1849, the *Lancet* – clearly excited by the sight-
ing of 'strange new bodies' – published an article by Swayne
describing the findings. So keen was the journal to rush its great
scoop into print that it didn't wait for the drawings to arrive but
published them separately in the following issue. 'These cells vary
very much in size and apparent structure during the different stages
of their development,' wrote Swayne.

The smallest are of the same size or even much less than blood
globules; so that to show them properly, an object-glass of high
magnifying power is required. They are very transparent and,
like blood discs, appear to be flattened cells; but the thickness of
their walls causes them to resemble rings in appearance. Their
interior is almost entirely destitute of granules. Their walls

refract light powerfully; they sometimes present a clotted or even cellular appearance, and there is usually a transverse figure or crack at some point of their circumference. In some of them I have observed very minute cells or buds project at different points of their circumferences ... The medium and large cells distinctly resemble the small cells in appearance but they are coarser and more granular in structure.

The same week William Budd set out both the results of his water analyses and the conclusions he had reached from them. Cholera, Budd argued, was caused by a living organism, seemingly some type of fungus, by which he meant a tiny parasite. Sharing Snow's belief that the cholera 'poison' had to be swallowed, Budd went on to say that when it reached the human gut it reproduced itself in huge numbers – reproduction being one of the characteristics of all life. And it was this action, he maintained, that caused the infamous massive discharges from the bowels which were so distinctive of the disease. These new organisms grew only in the human intestine, Budd believed. They spread as tiny particles in the air and in food, he thought, but their main route of transmission was through the drinking water in those areas where the disease was rife.

Budd then went on to make a surprising acknowledgement: 'As water is the principal channel through which this poison finds its way into the human body – a fact already established by the researches of Dr Snow, and of the discovery of which he must have all the whole merit – so is procuring pure water for drink the first and most effectual means of preventing its action.' Budd, who had a special interest in the spread of epidemic disease, had not only read Snow's work then but, virtually alone among his medical colleagues, had been impressed. Now with the results of his own research, he was convinced.

The sensational revelation that huge numbers of a previously unknown species might swarm in the water and air wherever cholera was present fascinated doctors and public alike. Subsequently the theories about cholera being a water-borne disease were sidelined. Instead, the national press and the medical journals burst into stories, speculation and, of course, ill-tempered spats between doctors, much of which centred on whether or not the cells were fungi, as Budd believed. And some medical gentlemen were clearly keen to be associated with this apparent breakthrough. Mr Grove, for example, claimed to have seen the very same bodies in cholera patients' urine, while Dr Cowdell, physician to Dorset County hospital, announced that he had noticed identical particles in the victims' sweat.

Scientists had known about the existence of creatures so small that they could not be made out by the naked eye since 1674, when a Dutch clothmaker, Antony van Leeuwenhoek, first peered at a drop of puddle water through the magnifying lens that he had painstakingly ground out of glass and was hardly able to believe what he saw. He was looking at the first micro-organisms – Little Animals in Rain Water as he called them – ever to be seen by man. He wrote excitedly to the Royal Society in London the first in a long series of letters describing his extraordinary observations through his magical instrument, the microscope.

Not surprisingly, after these astounding results, the clothmaker soon moved on from puddles to studying virtually every liquid and surface he could think of, including his own teeth. 'My teeth are kept usually very clean, nevertheless when I view them in a magnifying glass I find growing between them a little white matter as thick as wetted flour,' he wrote. 'In this substance, though I did not perceive any motion, I judged there might probably be living creatures. I therefore took some of this flour and mixt it either with pure rain water wherein there were not animals, or else with some of my spittle, and to my great surprise perceived that the aforesaid matter contained very many small living animals, which moved themselves very extravagently.' He concluded: 'The number of animals in the scurf of a man's teeth are so many that I believe they exceed the number of men in a kingdom.'

This is Leeuwenhoek's description of what we now call bacteria:

There was a . . . sort, which were so small that I was not able to give them any figure at all. These were a thousand times smaller than the eye of a large louse . . . I have often observed them to stand still as it were on a point and then turn themselves about with that swiftness, as we see a top turn round, the circumference they made being no larger than that of a grain of small sand, and then extending themselves straight forward, and by and by lying in a bending posture.

He went on to describe various other types of mostly single-cell organisms, such as simple algae and fungi. Any firmly established link between Leeuwenhoek's animalcules, and disease and decay had to wait nearly two hundred years, although when Budd and his colleagues announced their discovery some progress had been made.

The germ theory of disease – that says that infection results from tiny, self-multiplying bodies that can be spread by direct or indirect contact with infected objects, such as clothing, or passed through the air over long distances – has a surprisingly long history. One hundred years before the birth of Christ, the Roman scholar Marcus Terentius Varro warned about the dangers of marshy places because 'certain minute animals grow there which the eye cannot detect, and which get inside the nostrils, and give rise to stubborn distempers'. Another proponent of the idea that disease was caused by tiny particles, and also that it was contagious, was the fifteenth-century doctor Girolamo Fracastoro, a colleague of the astronomer Nicolas Copernicus at Padua University, one of whose claims to fame was writing an epic poem of nearly 1,300 verses on the distinctly unpoetic subject of syphilis.

And in the eighteenth century an English physician called Benjamin Marten wrote a book about tuberculosis called *A New Theory of Consumptions*, in which he suggested: 'The original and essential cause [of many different conditions, including strokes, gout, plague and depression] may possibly be some certain species of animalcules, or wonderfully minute living creatures, that, by their peculiar shape or disagreeable parts, are inimicable to our nature but, however, capable of subsisting in our juices and vessels, and . . . may cause all the disorders that have been mentioned.' Dr Marten went on to speculate that there might be different species of animalcules, each responsible for a different disease, and also that each species might travel together in vast numbers, like shoals of fish or swarms of flying insects, which would explain why epidemics raged in a particular country at a particular time of the year.

In the early nineteenth century, work on what is known as the 'Blood of Christ' miracle had produced some unexpected and hotly contested findings, certainly as far as the Roman Catholic Church was concerned. In 1263, a priest celebrating Mass in the church of St Christina in Bolsena, Italy, had been awestruck when blood appeared to seep from the bread that he had just consecrated, trickle over his hands and drip on to the altar. The Church hailed this as a true miracle: God showing that the Host was indeed the very flesh of Jesus; and the then pope was moved to establish the feast of Corpus Christi in honour of the event. Yet the St Christina story was by no means unique, and other examples of red, blood-like spots appearing on moist bread and wafers – whether consecrated or not – were recorded from time to time. Over half a century later, an Italian called Bartholomeo Bizio looked at some of these spots under a microscope and saw what he called a fungus – the terms fungus and virus were often used interchangeably, and sometimes to describe what are now called bacteria. Bizio moistened some bread and polenta and left them in a warm, damp place. Twenty-four hours later, both substances were covered with a bright red growth. The organism that Bizio had seen was, in fact, *Serratia marcescens*, a bacterium once thought harmless but now known to be capable of causing infections such as meningitis in human beings.

And by the time Budd and his colleagues announced their great discovery, at least one micro-organism had already been firmly identified as the cause of a specific disease. In 1835, another

Italian, a government official and farmer called Agostino Bassi, had shown that the devastating muscardine disease in silkworms that threatened the entire silk industry was caused by a mould fungus, now named *Beauvaria bassiana*. After years of painstaking, frustrating work that sometimes led Bassi to weep with disappointment, and despite a constant struggle with failing eyesight, the dogged amateur scientist eventually managed to show that muscardine could be induced in a silkworm only through direct contact with the source of the infection. 'I carried out all possible experiments with the object of making muscardine arise spontaneously in the silk worm,' he wrote.

> I inflicted the cruellest treatment on them, and used several kinds of poisons; mineral, vegetable and animal. I employed irritant, corrosive and caustic substances; acids, alkalis, earths and metals. In short, the most noxious substances, deadly to the animal organism ... but everything proved useless for my purpose ... The organism that I am about to describe alone has the power of achieving this result [that is, causing muscardine]. This murderous creature is organic, living and vegetable, a parasite fungus.

While all the horrible substances that Bassi had inflicted upon his tortured silkworms had failed to produced the disease, so the infectious agent that he eventually identified succeeded every time. 'One can infect caterpillars artificially merely by touching them with the point of a needle [carrying the fungus], by touching the substance on which they feed or by pricking their skin with a pin after extracting the contagious principle from diseased insects or objects infected by them,' he observed. And this time, the organism concerned really was what is now termed a fungus, not a bacterium as Bizio's *Serratia marcescens* on the bread was eventually proved to be.

The term fungus is now used to describe a particular type of microorganism that lives off a massive range of hosts – plants, animals and human beings – often causing disease and death. Some feed on dead organic matter and are part of the process of decomposition. Once classified as plants partly because of their inability to move unaided, fungi lack the stem, root and leaf structure and the chlorophyll that characterise what is now defined as plant life. Yeasts, rusts, moulds, mushrooms and mildews are all types of fungi, as are the organisms responsible for human diseases such as thrush and ringworm.

By 1849, scientists were rightly speculating that one extraordinary fungus was responsible for both a sickness in human beings and a disease in a species of plant, although their suspicion was more the result of a lucky guess than careful experiment. The human condition is ergot poisoning, or ergotism, caused by the strange fungus, *Claviceps purpurea*. *Claviceps purpurea* infects rye and some other grains and releases a toxin. If human beings eat this infected grain then the result is ergot poisoning. One of *Claviceps purpurea*'s many effects on the human body is to make the uterus contract, and it was *Claviceps purpurea*, therefore, that Dr Locock prescribed in small medicinal doses for Queen Victoria in order to speed up the birth of Princess Beatrice, while John Snow stood by with the chloroform. A chemical derived from *Claviceps purpurea* is sometimes given today to induce labour, while another derivative is used to treat migraine.

Ergot in the wrong dose and the wrong form, however, is deadly, and can result in one of two horrible conditions, both potentially fatal. Convulsive ergotism, also known as St Anthony's Fire, causes violent shaking, burning sensations, bodily contortions, delusions and hallucinations. In fact, ergot is the source of lysergic acid diethulamide, or LSD. Small wonder then that before the disease was understood, its victims were thought to be possessed. A preacher described what happened to people during an epidemic in America in 1741: 'When they come out of their trances, they commonly tell a senseless story of heaven and hell and what they saw there . . . In some towns several persons, both men and women that formerly were sober and to all appearance truly pious, are raving distracted, so that they are confined and chained. Many fall into epilepsies as they walk in the streets.'

And a new theory about the famous case of the Salem witches in New England in the late seventeenth century – when nineteen people were hanged or crushed to death for supposedly trafficking with the devil – is that the tragedy was sparked by a mass outbreak of ergot poisoning. Those who were thought to have been bewitched showed the classic signs of ergotism: going into 'fits', having out-of-body experiences, suffering temporary blindness and speechlessness, and seeing visions.

One of the accusers of seventy-one-year-old Rebecca Nurse, who was executed on 19 July 1692, described the behaviour of one of Nurse's alleged victims in the week before he died: 'He was acting in a very strange maner with most violent fitts . . . and he died a most violent death with dreadfull fitts, and the doctor that was with him said he could not tell what his distemper was.'

Gangrenous ergotism, on the other hand, causes the blood vessels to constrict, cutting off the blood supply to the extremities and leading to the condition known as dry gangrene that can kill the toes, fingers, ear lobes or even arms and legs, causing them literally to drop off. Unlike convulsive ergotism – which is the acute form of ergot poisoning caused by a short-term, high dose – gangrenous ergotism comes from eating low doses over a long period. Frostbite is a better known cause of dry gangrene, although, of course, this is due to extreme cold and not poisoning. A nineteenth-century description of the symptoms of dry gangrene talks of 'a tingling numbness of the extremities, which soon begin to wither, becoming dry as touchwood, emaciated like the limbs of Egyptian mummies, and black and hard as if they had been charred. In this state, they drop off at the joints, the toes separating in the milder cases; the feet in severer attacks falling at the ankle joints; the legs at the knees and even the thighs at the hips.' One tragic outbreak recorded in the seventeenth century near Bury St Edmunds affected a poverty-stricken labourer and his wife and five children, who bought a bushel of diseased wheat every week to bake bread and cakes because it was so cheap. After several months on this diet, the whole family went down with gangrenous ergotism. Their physician, Dr Wollaston, reported the appalling outcome to the Royal Society:

Mary, the mother, aged 40: right foot off at the ankle; left leg mortified, a mere bone but not off

Elizabeth, aged 13, both legs off below the knee

Sarah, aged 10, one foot off at the ankle

Robert, aged 10, both legs off below the knee

Edward, aged 4, both feet off at the ankles

An infant, aged 4 months, dead

The father was attacked to a slighter degree. The pain was confined to two fingers of his right hand which blackened and withered.

By 1849, scientists were also fairly sure of a relationship between other fungi and some more commonplace plant diseases not dangerous to humans, like rust in roses and canker in soft fruit, although they were not entirely clear about the precise role of fungi: did the fungus always cause the disease – as Bassi had shown that the muscardine fungus killed the previously healthy silkworm – or sometimes merely seize their chance to invade and kill an already sickly plant?

When Budd made his claims, there had already been some speculation about fungi and cholera. In a pamphlet impressively named 'On the Cryptogamous Origin of Malarious and Epidemic Fevers', written in 1848, for example, one Dr Mitchell expressed himself struck by the white, yellow, grey and black moulds that stained garments, utensils and pavements, made the fogs foetid and caused disagreeable odours and spots, even in the recesses of closets and the interior of trunks and desks. 'The singular prevalence of malarious [feverish, epidemic] diseases in the autumn is best explained by the fungi which grow most commonly at the same season,' Dr Mitchell concluded.

And in 1832 in Oxford, while cholera was raging, a Dr Burnet had reported what he described as 'an abundant purpling of the ground, as if red wine or blood had been poured out'. In fact, this phenomenon, known as bloody rain, gory dew or red snow, is caused by various types of algae – a group of aquatic, plant-like organisms – that produce a bright red pigment, capable of dyeing ponds, cave walls and even entire mountain-sides, shades ranging from pale pink to brilliant crimson.

By 1849, such manifestations were no longer considered supernatural but they were wrongly thought to be fungoid in origin and perhaps linked to epidemics. Sometimes when cholera was at large, 'the ground has been seen to redden, as if the earth were sweating blood, the rain has fallen in drops of the same sinister hue, and the ponds and tanks resemble pools of gore,' one observer declared, clearly suspecting a link between the two events. In fact, the timing was pure coincidence. The subject that was to become the modern science of microbiology was largely shrouded in confusion, but by the mid-1800s scientists and philosophers had come to realise, first, that there was an association between 'animalcules' and putrefaction in organic matter, and, second, that there was an association between 'animalcules' and specific diseases in animals and plants.

Much of this knowledge had come about because of man's struggle to answer one of the most fundamental questions posed by natural science; namely, what is it that sparks life itself?

One theory of the origins of life that enjoyed widespread support for hundreds of years was that of spontaneous generation. The Greek philosopher Aristotle, in the fourth century BC, was among those to espouse it, and in the mid-nineteenth century it still had some adherents, although by then its days were seriously numbered.

Spontaneous generation held that some life forms arose spontaneously from non-living matter, particularly when that matter was decaying. People had noticed, for example, that fungi grew on rotting wood, that maggots wriggled in putrid flesh and that wasps sometimes lived in the carcasses of dead animals, and they thought that these species must have arisen directly out of their host or habitat. A seventeenth-century recipe for producing mice recommended placing dirty underwear and husks of wheat together in a jar so that the sweat from the underwear would penetrate the husks, thus changing them into mice. The process was said to take about three weeks.

Some of the most exotic stories about spontaneous generation had much in common with ancient legends and religious beliefs, such as the idea of a phoenix rising from the ashes. The fifteenth-century scholar Julius Caesar Scaliger wrote to a friend: 'You may rather wonder that in the Britannick Ocean a bird unknown in your parts hangs by the beak in the timber of rotten ships till it grow to perfection and swim away, being fashioned like a duck, and living upon filth. I have also seen one of these fowls.' And he also described a shellfish 'as it seemed not very large, in which there was a young bird almost perfected, with the tops of the wings, the bill and the feet sticking to the farthest parts of the shell'. The barnacle goose takes its name from this legend.

Scaliger's contemporary, the Jewish doctor Amatus Lusitanus, proved more sceptical about a dramatic example of spontaneous generation, however. 'I have heard here in England strange stories of people that have had wolves in their flesh which they were fain to feed daily with raw beef, which I allwaies reckoned for fables,' he recounted. 'I know a woman in Amsterdam that pretended one in her brest, but upon visitation I found it an imposture to move pity, that the meat which was given her to feed the wolf she might eat herself.'

Then in 1668, the Italian physician and poet, Francesco Redi, a contemporary of Leeuwenhoek, succeeded in demonstrating that maggots came from flies' eggs, rather than arising spontaneously from rotting meat as was generally believed: 'Although it be a matter of daily observation that infinite numbers of worms are produced in dead bodies and decayed plants, I feel inclined to believe that these worms are all generated by insemination, and that putrefied matter in which they are found has no other office than that of serving as a place or suitable nest where animals deposit their eggs at the breeding season, and in which they also find nourishment.' To prove his point, he put portions of meat into flasks; some open to the air, some sealed completely and some covered with gauze. As he expected, maggots appeared only in the open flasks where the flies were able to reach the meat and lay their eggs. This type of experiment, which uses comparisons – known as controls – as yardsticks against which to assess the results, remains the gold standard for scientific research.

And Leeuwenhoek's studies of minute life also provided powerful evidence against spontaneous generation – for example, by showing that weevils found in wheat were hatched from the eggs of flying insects, not bred from the wheat itself, and that shellfish were spawned, not produced out of mud or sand. Leeuwenhoek would walk around the streets of Delft, his pockets bulging with larvae and pupae hatching out in glass tubes, while families of lice bred in his stockings, allowed to feed on his feet in order that he might study their lifecycle. To prove his point about reproduction, he also made drawings of the penis of the grain weevil and the testicles of the flea based on his observations through a microscope.

Still not everyone was convinced, and in 1745, an English clergyman called John Turbevill Needham designed an experiment that he claimed would settle the matter once and for all. By then, it was believed that all micro-organisms were killed by boiling (this is true for the vast majority, although not all). 'For my purpose, therefore, I took a quantity of mutton gravy, hot from the fire,' Needham explained. He reasoned that the boiled broth would now contain no live organisms, and he proceeded to seal it in a flask and wait. When he re-opened the bottle: 'My phial swarmed with life, and with microscopic animals of most dimensions, from some of the largest I had ever seen to some of the least. The very first drop I used upon opening it yielded me multitudes, perfectly formed, animated and spontaneous in all their motions.'

This appearance of live organisms in sterile broth led Needham to claim victory for spontaneous generation, but another cleric, an Italian priest called Lazzaro Spallanzani, wondered if perhaps the organisms had found their way into the broth from the air after the liquid had been boiled. To test this, Spallanzani put broth into a sealed flask and first drew off the air to create a vacuum before boiling and storing it. When Spallanzani's flask was re-opened, no micro-organisms were to be found. His critics, however, said that all he had proved was that spontaneous generation needed air in order to work. The arguments would only finally be consigned to history in 1859 when the French chemist, Louis Pasteur, used a more sophisticated version of Needham's and Spallanzani's experiments to dispose of spontaneous generation once and for all.

In the pre-Pasteur world of 1849, however, opinions about the composition and nature of micro-organisms and their possible role in disease and decay were still varied and confused. Among the ideas to enjoy a burst of popularity were those of the German chemist Justus von Liebig, who suggested that decay was a chemical not a biological process; in other words, the 'germs' or particles that caused putrefaction were not themselves alive, and the living organisms that were seen on rotting material were like vultures, merely feeding off a corpse, and not themselves responsible for the death. John Snow was among those to profess an interest in Liebig's theory.

Against this background then, the Bristol doctors announced their findings, but William Budd's claims that the new 'cholera cells' were a type of fungus added an extra level of confusion to the events that followed and were to lead to the group's downfall. The first substantive doubts were cast when George Busk, president of the Microscopical Society of London, announced the results of his attempts to see the same bodies in the discharges of cholera patients. He could find nothing remotely like Budd and Swayne had described in his samples, he said, and his guess was that their so-called cholera cells were in reality grains of starch, pieces of corn husk and 'uredos', or spores, from the organism that caused the disease wheat rust and commonly found in bread. There was certainly no new type of fungus, Busk was sure.

Meanwhile, the Royal College of Physicians had also been looking into the Bristol claims and on the same day that Busk presented his findings, William Baly and William Gull delivered the college's verdict. First, they had not been able to find these bodies in either air or water, including in a sample of water from a tank at Albion Terrace supplied to them by John Snow, perhaps in the hope that they would take his theory seriously. Second, they said, the Bristol team seemed to be confusing the many very different bodies present in cholera discharges, most of which could be traced to the food or medicine that the patients had consumed, and, while it was not clear where the remainder came from, they were certainly not fungi. And what was more, all of the most distinctive cells were to be found in specimens from people with very different diseases to cholera.

The final conclusion left no one in any doubt about how the gentlemen from the Royal College regarded any so-called breakthrough: 'We draw from these premises, bodies found and described by Messrs Brittan and Swayne are not the cause of cholera and have no exclusive connection with that disease; or, in other words, that the whole theory of the disease which has recently been propounded is erroneous as far as it is based on the existence of the bodies in question.'

And that, it seemed, was that. Despite the *Lancet*'s almost mandatory rubbishing of the College's report – calling it 'somewhat twaddling', and mocking one of the contributors for 'collecting cobwebs and scraping broken glass in St Giles [one of London's most notorious slums]' in his attempt to find the elusive cholera cells – the views of the Royal College of Physicians were generally accepted as conclusive.

At the end of October, James Paget, one of the surgeons for whom Snow was to administer anaesthesia, wrote to a relative who was keen to follow up the findings for himself:

I could not today obtain any cholera fungi for you, but I will try to do so tomorrow again. I believe, however, that the whole hypothesis will shortly be exploded, for it appears certain that many of the things seen are not fungi but remnants of food taken; that they are to be found in cases of typhus and dysentery and some other diseases, and that they are not to be found in the air or water of many of the worst cholera districts. All recent examinations except at Bristol are, I am told, opposed to the fungus theory.

Budd and his colleagues did not fight back but appear to have dropped the matter fast once the doubts began to be expressed. The Bristol affair turned out to be one of those overnight sensations that are as quickly forgotten in the cold light of day. And with the fungus theory condemned, no one who mattered paid much heed to the idea that cholera might be caused by some other, non-fungoid, type of 'germ' in the digestive system, nor to Budd's endorsement of Snow's view that the disease was mainly waterborne and that people needed only to wash their hands thoroughly and drink clean water to avoid infection. The chance to save tens of thousands of lives was missed once again.

John Snow took no part in the great fungus debate. He was not a microscopist and his interests lay elsewhere. He wanted to know how cholera behaved within the body and how it was spread from one person to another – the precise nature of any organism involved did not seem to concern him. That October, he gave a talk at the Western Literary Institution in which he referred to the Bristol claims but while he clearly found them worth mentioning, he stopped well short of endorsing them. So, when the fungus theory was dismissed and the work of Budd, Swayne and Brittan with it, Snow at least emerged unscathed, although still largely ignored.

Exactly what it was that Budd and his colleagues found remains a mystery to this day. The chances are that the doctors were indeed

mistaken, although whether they were looking at fragments of par-
tially digested food, at human cells or at some other insignificant
type of particle, no one knows. But it is just possible that, in the
discharges and the water supply at least, the Bristol three had stumbled upon that elusive agent that had been wreaking destruction
across the world for more than thirty years. If so, their great discovery ended in ignominy, partly at least because they called it by
the wrong name.

CHAPTER 10

The Grand Experiment

It is beyond dispute that ... a portion of the inhabitants of the metropolis are made to consume in some form or other, a portion of their own excrement and, moreover, to pay for the privilege

Arthur Hill Hassall, microscopist, 1850

It was a brave soul who drank a glass of water in Britain's towns and cities in the first half of the nineteenth century. Anyone who did opt to play Russian roulette with their health in this way obtained the noxious stuff from a variety of sources – from streams and rivers, from wells and from standpipes in the street. Some had it piped direct to their homes, like the unfortunate residents of Albion Terrace. But whatever its source, most water was disgusting and dangerous – a cloudy brew of slime, industrial effluent and the recycled waste products of people's bowels.

By the 1840s, London's water supplies were in the greedy grasp of private companies, most of whom took their product straight from the Thames in the middle of the capital – near the spot where the sewage from three million inhabitants was disgorged to lap gently to and fro with the tide – and pumped it out, untreated, direct to their customers. When the microscopist Arthur Hill Hassall examined samples from two water companies, which they insisted had been filtered, he found 'the hairs of animals and numerous substances which had passed through the alimentary canal'.

Matters were made much worse in 1848 when Edwin Chadwick, in a well-meaning attempt to stop the capital's poor from floundering in their own excrement, speeded up a move to take cesspools out of use and flush the sewers into the Thames. In January that year he announced that 'the evil of sending refuse down into the Thames was utterly inconsiderable compared with the evil of keeping accumulations of noxious matter in densely inhabited localities'. From March to May then, 29,000 cubic yards of filth were deposited in the river, followed by a further 80,000 cubic yards from September to the following February. Six years later, all household and street refuse was being tipped into the Thames, while 30,000 cesspools had been abolished, according to the engineer Joseph Bazalgette. And there were powerful forces lined up against any attempt to make the water companies clean up their act. After all, huge profits were being made, and in the early 1850s the government found itself in difficulties when it tried to introduce some modest reforms: eighty-six MPs turned out to be water company shareholders.

The scientist Michael Faraday complained to *The Times* about a stomach-churning trip down the river one hot July day in the 1850s.

> I traversed this day by steam-boat the space between London and Hungerford Bridges; it was low water, and I think the tide must have been near the turn. The appearance and the smell of the water forced themselves at once on my attention. The whole of the river was an opaque pale brown fluid. In order to test the degree of opacity, I tore up some white cards into pieces, moistened them so as to make them sink easily below the surface, and then dropped some of these pieces into the water at every pier; before they had sunk an inch below the surface they were indistinguishable, though the sun shone brightly at the time; and when the pieces fell edgeways, the lower part was hidden from

sight before the upper part was under water. This happened at St Paul's Wharf, Blackfriars Bridge, Temple Wharf, Southwark Bridge, and Hungerford; and I have no doubt would have occurred further up and down the river. Near the bridges, the feculence rolled up in clouds so dense that they were visible at the surface, even in water of this kind.

The smell was very bad, and common to the whole of the water; it was the same as that which now comes up from the gully-holes in the streets; the whole river was for the time a real sewer. Having just returned from out of the country air, I was, perhaps, more affected by it than others, but I do not think I could have gone on to Lambeth or Chelsea . . .

When the country's second and most terrible cholera epidemic finally petered out in late 1849 after killing 52,000 people, John Snow was thirty-six and still living at 54 Frith Street in Soho. By now he was busily building up his anaesthesia practice and spending much of his spare time on his research into sleep-inducing gases. If he was at all put out at the reception given to his cholera pamphlet, he characteristically kept his feelings to himself, and certainly any disappointment that he might have felt had no apparent effect on his determination to carry on with his cholera research. Over the next five years, he continued to collect evidence from national statistics, local reports and personal accounts from doctors who had been involved in both British and foreign outbreaks, examining how each local outbreak had started, its pattern of spread, how the victims had lived and, most important to him, the source and quality of the local water supply.

In 1853, John Snow was finally given some measure of official recognition by being mentioned in a report by William Baly and William Gull of the Royal College of Physicians. In 1849, Baly and Gull had dismissed the claims of William Budd and his colleagues in Bristol, and the pair now turned their attention to some of the other ideas about the causes and spread of cholera. Encouragingly they had at least heard of Snow, although their opening remarks did not bode well: at first glance his theory had 'the aspect of great improbability', Baly and Gull thought, but they did at least discuss that theory before going on to condemn it as 'untenable'. Their main objection was that not everyone who developed cholera seemed to live near a source of contaminated drinking water, and they concluded that good ventilation was the best weapon in the fight against the disease.

Snow took Baly and Gull in his stride, merely commenting some time later that they had done him the honour of giving him a fair hearing. Honour aside though, John Snow was no more swayed by

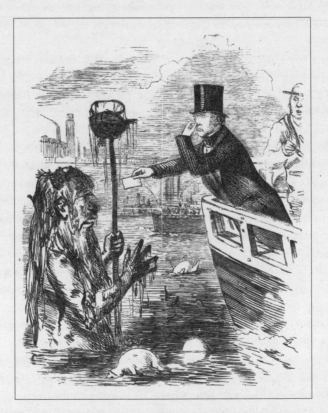

Michael Faraday dropping pieces of card into the Thames,
as depicted by a *Punch* cartoonist

the views of the Royal College of Physicians than the College had been by him: all the material he had found to date served only to convince him even more that he was right. Occasionally during the years 1851–3 when he came upon another account of a cholera outbreak that he thought provided a particularly strong piece of supporting evidence for his theory, he wrote it up as an academic paper, published largely in the *London Medical Gazette*. But as usual there was no discernible reaction from the medical profession. What Snow really needed was a method of putting his theory properly to the test by means of a scientific experiment. Five years after his first tentative venture into the public domain on the subject of cholera, the reappearance of the disease showed him the way forward.

Seventeen years had passed between Britain's first cholera epidemic in 1831 and its second. The next time it was back sooner. In the summer of 1853, in a sickeningly familiar pattern, the disease was again at the Baltic ports. All of Britain now knew what would happen next: it was just a matter of when and where. The Treasury turned down Chadwick's request to send a medical officer to Hamburg to 'watch the progress of the disease', presumably on the grounds that the medical officer in question would, in just a few days, be able to watch the progress of the disease on the British side of the North Sea, thus saving taxpayers the cost of his fare. On 3 September, a letter arrived in Whitehall from a Dr Robinson reporting a fatal case of Asiatic cholera in Newcastle. By 12 September, Richard Grainger, like Dr Daun more than twenty years before him, had been despatched to the city, and was reporting seventy-three new cases in the space of one weekend and twenty-seven deaths. Four days later, he was telegraphing Chadwick asking for a team of doctors to help him.

The epidemic that winter was largely confined to north-east England, but a lull in the spring was followed by a renewed assault in the summer of 1854, and now it was London's turn to suffer. The story has it that the capital's troubles began when the chief mate of a ship just docked from the Baltic brought the soiled linen of a sick officer ashore for washing. Soon after, London saw its first cases of cholera, mainly among people involved in shipping on the river.

South London had suffered particularly badly in the 1848–9 outbreak and Snow was sure he knew why. Water here was largely provided by two companies, the Lambeth Water Company and the Southwark and Vauxhall, and until the early 1850s both drew their supplies from the most polluted part of the river. Some parts of south London were supplied by one company and some by the other, but there was also a third area where the two companies were in competition, their pipes running together down the streets and into the courts and alleys. In consequence, one household often had a different supply from its next-door neighbour.

In 1849, it had mattered little which company the householder chose, for the supplies were equally revolting, but in 1852 the Lambeth Water Company had moved their works from opposite Hungerford Market in central London, now the site of Charing Cross station, up the Thames Valley to rural Thames Ditton, where the Thames is no longer tidal and therefore well out of reach of the capital's filthy outpourings. Southwark and Vauxhall continued merrily as before.

So in 1854 when the victims started dying once again on the south bank of the Thames, Snow realised that here, set out before him, was the perfect, ready-made natural experiment. He would compare the numbers of victims whose water was supplied by the two different companies during the 1848–9 epidemic, before Lambeth's 'clean up', with the numbers of victims supplied by the two companies in this present epidemic. According to his theory, the resulting statistics should show that sewage-free drinking water meant fewer deaths from cholera.

And in the district with the mixed supply, the miasmatists wouldn't be able to claim that one group lived in cleaner houses with fewer smells because he would be comparing like with like. 'As there is no difference whatever, either in the houses or the people receiving the supply of the two water companies, or in any of the physical conditions with which they are surrounded, it is obvious that no experiment could have been devised which would more thoroughly test the effect of the water supply on the progress of cholera than this,' he wrote. 'Three hundred thousand people of both sexes, of every age and occupation, and of every rank and station, from gentlefolk to the very poor, were divided into two groups without their choice, and, in most cases, without their knowledge; one group being supplied with water containing the sewage of London, and, amongst it, whatever might have come from the cholera patients, the other group having water quite free from such impurity.'

What is now known as Snow's 'Grand Experiment' is a classic study in the science of epidemiology that is still analysed and debated today, and John Snow is often referred to as the father of epidemiology because of it. Epidemiologists work in the field of public health – in other words, they are concerned with the health of populations rather than with individual patients. The zealous Edwin Chadwick was mistaken about the causes of contagious epidemic disease, and he wasn't a doctor, but he was nevertheless a leading figure in public health because he recognised the vital importance of hygiene, albeit for the wrong reasons.

By the end of the nineteenth century, the sanitary movement as it became known, of which Charles Dickens was a leading light, had succeeded in forcing the authorities to provide clean streets, efficient sewers and safe drinking water.

A dictionary definition of epidemiology is 'that branch of medical science which treats epidemics', and the term 'epidemic' is used to describe what happens when a disease attacks many people suddenly and simultaneously. It is usually also associated with rapid and unpleasant deaths on a large scale. The term comes from the Greek 'epi' meaning 'upon', and 'demos' meaning the people or the mob: literally, the disease falls upon the masses. An epidemic then is episodic and occurs at a particular time and place, although the term is used today to cover outbreaks of very different durations and extent; lung cancer as well as influenza, for example.

An often quoted description of epidemiology is 'the study of the distribution and determinants of health-related states or events in a specified population, and the application of this study to the control of health problems'. Distribution in this context means the analysis by time, place and classes of people affected. Determinants are all the physical, biological, social, cultural and behavioural factors that have an impact on health. Health-related states and events include diseases, the causes of death, behaviour such as smoking and use of the health services.

Put simply, epidemiology is concerned with two questions: who gets sick and why? And because epidemiologists' work involves the piecing together of evidence in order to 'solve' the mystery of a new disease or an unusual outbreak of a known disease, they are called the medical detectives. They collect and study a massive amount of data to try to determine who is most at risk from a particular disease or condition, and where, how and when the victims were exposed, which means that statistics and disease 'mapping' are vital tools. One of the axioms of epidemiology is that a disease is distributed not at random but according to a web of complicated and often inter-connected factors. For an individual, some of these risk factors could be congenital – that is, a predisposition to a particular disease could be inherited – while others might be due to lifestyle, for example, a bad diet or smoking, or they could be based on age or gender, such as cancer and heart disease. But epidemiologists also look at many risk factors that are not related to the individual but environmental, linked to those places and times of the year where and when the disease is prevalent.

In 400 BC, the Greek physician Hippocrates, perhaps the most famous figure in the Western tradition of medicine, wrote a treatise called 'On Airs, Waters, and Places' in which he stressed the importance of geography, climate and the seasons in matters of health and sickness.

Whoever wishes to investigate medicine properly, should proceed thus: in the first place to consider the seasons of the year, and what effects each of them produces ... Then the winds, the hot and the cold, especially such as are common to all countries, and then such as are peculiar to each locality . . . In the same manner, when one comes into a city to which he is a stranger, he ought to consider its situation, how it lies as to the winds and the rising of the sun . . . And concerning the waters which the inhabitants use, whether they be marshy and soft, or hard and running from elevated and rocky situations, and then if saltish and unfit for cooking; and the ground, whether it be naked and deficient in water, or wooded and well watered, and whether it lies in a hollow, confined situation, or is elevated and cold.

From these things he must proceed to investigate everything else. For if one knows all these things well . . . he cannot miss knowing, when he comes into a strange city, either the diseases peculiar to the place, or the particular nature of common diseases, so that he will not be in doubt as to the treatment of the diseases, or commit mistakes. And in particular, as the season and the year advances, he can tell what epidemic diseases will attack the city, either in summer or in winter, and what each individual will be in danger of experiencing from the change of regimen . . . Having made these investigations, and knowing beforehand the seasons, such a one must . . . succeed in the preservation of health, and be by no means unsuccessful in the practice of his art.

As Hippocrates implies, because epidemiology looks at the causes of disease and at risk factors, it plays an important part in preventive medicine: providing information and strategies, both for individuals and for governments, to try to stop disease gaining hold.

Another key aspect of epidemiology that distinguishes it from other medical sciences is that its studies are conducted across human populations in the field. Animal experiments in the laboratory allow researchers to have complete control over the environment and over their subjects' exposure to a particular chemical, drug or pathogen, but the resulting findings may not turn out to be in any way applicable to human beings; and scientists have no way of predicting how relevant the findings for one species will be to another, if at all. There are constant surprises about the differences and also the similarities between humans and various species of animal life. 'Who could have guessed that homo sapiens would share with the humble guinea pig the unenviable distinction of being incapable of synthesising ascorbic acid [vitamin C], or share with armadillos a susceptibility to the bacterium that causes leprosy, or that intestinal cancer usually occurs in the large intestine of humans and the small intestine of sheep?' wondered one researcher, grappling with the problem in the twentieth century.

And laboratory tests can bear little relation to what happens in the real world. For example, permanent hair dyes have been linked to certain types of cancers, but because the animals used in the research were fed huge doses of the dye into their stomachs throughout their lives, this may be of no help in estimating the risk posed to human beings who occasionally apply a small amount of the chemicals to their scalps. Animal research sometimes helps to explain why a particular substance causes or prevents a disease, but only epidemiology's straightforward observation of what actually happens in human populations allows the risks to human beings to be quantified in a meaningful way and action to be taken to reduce that risk.

In fact, epidemiology has often exposed dangers to health long before those dangers were understood. When Snow's colleagues did start to discuss his cholera theory, one of their criticisms was that he was unable to specify the precise nature of the cholera 'poison'. In 1849, an attempt to do just that had led to William Budd's work being badly discredited. Yet by concentrating on cholera's mode of transmission – which could only be done in the field – Snow made a greater contribution to public health than if he had sat in a laboratory and identified the agent responsible for the disease. One hundred years later, people were being warned that smoking caused lung cancer, although no one then, or now, understood the process involved. The public were, nevertheless, told of the dangers because epidemiology had highlighted the risks beyond all doubt. In the same way, a new type of tampon was identified as responsible for a large increase in toxic shock syndrome among young women and taken off the market, well before the precise mechanism involved could be explained.

In its early days, epidemiology was concerned solely with communicable diseases, but it is now concerned with a huge range of conditions, including cancers, heart disease and diabetes; and governments and bodies such as the World Health Organization look to epidemiology to find ways of preventing and controlling diseases, and to help plan health services and health education. The work is particularly vital as international travel causes the world to shrink, and diseases that have always been confined to one particular region start to spread, like cholera in the nineteenth century.

As John Snow pondered how to design an experiment based on the water supplies and the cholera deaths in south London that would give him the statistics to prove his theory, another doctor had compared like-for-like groups of people in a like-for-like situation, as Snow needed to do, in order to discover how a disease was being spread. This work had been on a smaller, more manageable scale, however, than the research that Snow was planning. The doctor concerned was a Hungarian, Ignaz Semmelweis, whose name is often linked with that of John Snow as an epidemiological pioneer.

In the early 1840s Semmelweis was working on a maternity ward at the General Hospital in Vienna; it was a well-known fact that the death rates for puerperal fever on Semmelweis's ward were three times higher than those on the hospital's other maternity ward. The women were admitted to one of the two wards at random, based on the day of the week they came in, so there were no obvious differences between them, for example in their general health or socio-economic class. Other people before Semmelweis, in particular the English doctors Charles White in Manchester and Robert Storrs in Yorkshire, had correctly hypothesised about the nature of puerperal fever and how it was being spread, although their message, like Snow's on cholera, was largely ignored.

Semmelweis is famous among epidemiologists then, not so much for the originality of his findings, as for the statistical, scientific approach that he brought to investigating the problem.

Puerperal fever, also known as childbirth fever, childbed fever or postpartum fever, occurs when a woman's uterus or vagina becomes infected with the bacterium *Streptococcus pyogenes*, usually within the first ten days after the baby is born. *Streptococcus pyogenes* is also responsible for a wide range of other diseases in humans, including scarlet fever and impetigo. If the localised genital infection then passes into the woman's bloodstream causing septicaemia, the condition can be deadly, and puerperal fever was a major killer of new mothers in the seventeenth, eighteenth and nineteenth centuries.

Semmelweis became obsessed with trying to discover the reason for the vastly different death rates on the two hospital wards. Again like Snow with cholera, he first looked at the pathology of the disease for clues as to its likely route of entry into the body and its mode of attack. He decided that puerperal fever must be a form of septicaemia, or blood poisoning, after noticing the similarity between the pathological findings for the infected mothers and those of one of his colleagues, who died when a knife wound received while carrying out a post-mortem became infected and turned to septicaemia. Semmelweis then wondered whether doctors and medical students might themselves be responsible for spreading puerperal fever because of their habit of coming straight from cutting up dead bodies to carrying out internal examinations on newly delivered women, either washing their hands very hastily between the two procedures or not washing them at all. The maternity ward with the low death rates was staffed by midwives who did no post-mortems.

How much, if anything, Semmelweis knew about the work of people like White and Storrs is not clear. But his contribution was that, having raised the hypothesis about how the fever was spread, he then set about testing it by comparing a range of factors. The patients on the two wards were from similar social and economic backgrounds, and one group was no sicker than the other. On the wards where they were being nursed, the ventilation, hygiene, crowding, food and drugs prescribed were the same. In fact, Semmelweis could find no significant differences anywhere. He began to pay special attention to the way that he himself practised medicine on his ward, doing examinations and operations very carefully, but women continued to die in large numbers.

Finally, having eliminated all other possible explanations to his satisfaction, he insisted that doctors scrubbed their hands with soap and water and then soaked them in chloride before carrying out pelvic examinations. Within seven months, puerperal fever deaths on Semmelweis's ward had plummeted from 120 per 1,000 births to 12 per 1,000, actually dipping below those on the mid-wives' ward. When he realised the truth, Semmelweis was tortured by the thought of his own past role in spreading the disease: 'Puerperal fever is caused by conveyance to the pregnant woman of putrid particles derived from living organisms through the agency of the examining fingers,' he wrote. 'Consequently must I make my confession that God only knows the number of women whom I have consigned prematurely to the grave.'

In the summer of 1854, John Snow resolved to spare no effort to 'crack' cholera, once and for all. And he decided to do the leg work himself so that he would have the whole satisfaction of uncovering the truth, one way or the other. Personally he needed no more convincing, but he knew his ideas to be so original and their implications for public health so huge that no doubts must remain. 'The circumstance of the cholera-poison passing down the sewers into a great river, and being distributed through miles of pipes and yet producing its specific effects, was a fact of so startling a nature and of so vast an importance to the community that it could not be too rigidly examined or established on too firm a basis,' he explained.

The Government's chief statistician, William Farr, was already col-lecting weekly returns of cholera deaths, broken down by sub-district, and so discovering the victims' addresses presented Snow with little problem. What did take time was finding out which house was supplied by which water company in the 'mixed supply' areas. For this, Snow set off on a quest of a type now known as 'shoe leather' epidemiology. Armed with his list of addresses where deaths had occurred, he travelled to south London and, like a detective solving a crime, he began weeks of pounding the streets and knocking on doors, asking the same question – from which company did the household get its water?

It was a frustrating business. 'There were very few instances in which I could at once get the information I required,' he explained. 'Even when the water-rates are paid by the residents, they can seldom remember the name of the water company till they have looked for the receipt. In the case of working people who pay weekly rents, the rates are invariably paid by the landlord or his agent, who often lives at a distance, and the residents know nothing about the matter.' This difficulty might well have scuppered the whole plan but Snow, as usual, was not to be beaten and he found an imaginative way around the problem. He discovered that the amount of salt in the two companies' water differed enormously and realised that this fact could be used to identify the supplier. 'It would, indeed, have been almost impossible for me to complete the inquiry, if I had not found that I could distinguish the water of the two companies with perfect certainty by a chemical test,' he wrote.

The chemical test involved adding a solution of silver nitrate to a sample of water and measuring the resulting amount of chloride of silver in the water, from which it was then possible to calculate the salt content. Snow found that the Lambeth water contained 0.95 grains of salt per gallon, while the Southwark and Vauxhall water contained an astounding 37.9 grains per gallon. In fact, the difference was such that it was possible to tell which water was which merely by adding the silver nitrate: the much greater levels of white silver chloride in the Southwark and Vauxhall water must have been clearly visible. Snow explained:

When the resident could not give clear and conclusive evidence about the water company, I obtained some of the water in a small phial, and wrote the address on the cover, when I could examine it after coming home. The mere appearance of the water generally afforded a very good indication of its source, especially if it was observed as it came in, before it had entered the water-butt or cistern; and the time of its coming in also afforded some evidence of the kind of water, after I had ascertained the hours when the turncocks of both companies visited any street. These points were, however, not relied on, except as corroborating more decisive proof, such as the chemical test or the company's receipt for the rates.

There was just one flaw in this: the salt test was based on a wrong premise. Snow thought that the high salt content of the Southwark and Vauxhall water was caused by sewage pollution, but he later learnt from one of the company's engineers that the salt was in fact due to a tidal backflow into the Thames from the North Sea and that this, in turn, depended on the climate. Inner London is much closer to the sea than the upper reaches of the Thames where Lambeth was by then taking its water. Luckily for Snow, while he was carrying out his research the weather stayed exceptionally hot and dry, which meant that the Southwark and Vauxhall salt content remained consistently high, thus ensuring that his method was reliable throughout the experiment. He later admitted that he had been fortunate: 'Throughout all the dry weather, which lasted while my enquiries were being made, a mixture of the sea water extended farther up the Thames than usual.'

The size of the task that Snow had set himself proved formidable and, despite driving himself non-stop, he was eventually forced to take on some help in the person of a local apothecary called John Joseph Whiting. Whiting carried out some of the door-to-door inquiries in Bermondsey, Rotherhithe and Wandsworth, and earned Snow's approval for the pains that he took with the work.

Finally, spurred on by the steady piling up of figures in his favour, and after some considerable number-crunching, in the late summer of 1854 Snow was ready to release his results. They came down to this: while in 1848–9 death rates from cholera had been equally high for the customers of both companies, by 1854 the mortality rate for people living in houses supplied by Southwark and Vauxhall was between eight and nine times higher than that for the houses with the clean Lambeth water.

In the first seven weeks of the 1854 epidemic, for example, in 40,046 Southwark and Vauxhall houses, there were 1, 263 cholera deaths, a rate of 315 per 10,000 houses. In 26,107 Lambeth houses, however, the deaths were 98, or 37 per 10,000 houses. And in the first four weeks of the epidemic, the figures were even more dramatic: 286 deaths for Southwark and Vauxhall and 14 for Lambeth, giving a fourteen-fold higher risk for the Southwark and Vauxhall customers. In fact, during those four weeks ending on 5 August, there had been only 563 deaths from cholera in the whole of London, and over half were of people supplied by the Southwark and Vauxhall water company, while many of the other deaths were of sailors and other people working on the Thames who took their water straight from the river.

This 'Grand Experiment' was the first major attempt to bring an ordered scientific approach to understanding how a disease is propagated and how it is spread or distributed within a population; and there in Snow's hands was now the proof that he had known all along must exist. For the first time, one of the countless cholera theories to be put forward since 1817, when the disease for no known reason began its trek across the world, had been subjected to a rigorous scientific analysis, and had passed with flying colours. At last, it seemed, Snow was about to unveil some findings that the good and the great of the medical profession would no longer be able to ignore. All he had to do now was to put the finishing touches to his research, write up his results and dig into his pockets to pay a printer.

Yet just as John Snow was preparing to release his discovery of a lifetime, something happened – something that caused him to stop in his tracks, to leave his foot-slogging through the lanes and yards of south London, and rush back home to the streets of Soho. An extraordinary drama was unfolding, literally on his doorstep, with which his name was to be linked for ever.

CHAPTER 11

A Plague on their Houses

The minds of those we saw were probably affected by the state of things around them. We had to obtain our information from persons whose friends and relatives were scarcely yet buried

David Fraser and Thomas Hughes, government inspectors,
Soho, September 1854

Dr Rogers had no hesitation about the death certificate. Reaching for the form, he wrote 'diarrhoea and exhaustion' in the column headed 'Cause of death'. He had seen more cases like this than he cared to count, and the child had been sickly from birth. The mother, poor wretch, was in a bad way too, and on one of his frequent visits to the ailing baby she had collapsed in front of him.

He knew the Lewis family well. They were respectable, hardworking people struggling to live a decent life in that part of Soho: the parents and baby together with two older children, aged eight and thirteen, were crammed into one ground-floor room at the back of a house at number 40 Broad Street, the other side of Oxford Street to Rogers' practice in Berners Street. When the wind was in the wrong direction, the smell from a neighbouring privy hung around the Lewis house like a fog.

William Rogers had been called out to forty-year-old Sarah Lewis several times during what had proved to be a troublesome fourth pregnancy, and he had been surprised and relieved when the birth itself turned out to be quite straightforward. But then Sarah had had no breast milk, which was always a bad sign for the infant. Cow's milk and rice were poor substitutes for mother's milk, and the Lewis baby's constant bouts of diarrhoea and vomiting over the weeks to come were absolutely typical. It was exactly what had happened four years earlier with the couple's previous child, Rogers remembered. That one, a boy, had had problems with his lungs as well as with his stomach, and had died at ten months. This new baby had survived for only five. Rogers had done what he could for her – which really wasn't that much – but then he had known all along that the case was probably hopeless. At eleven o'clock on the morning of Saturday 2 September her little frame had quietly given up what had never been a fair fight.

But this was no time for reflection about the Lewises or anyone else for that matter, for Rogers now found himself caught up in an emergency the like of which he had never seen, or expected to see, in his life.

It began on the night of Thursday 31 August 1854, three days after Sarah Lewis's baby fell ill for the last time. It had been a terrible day; the sky was yellow and glowering, the heat insufferable and the air not fit to breathe. The temperature climbed remorselessly to 98.5, and as the hours dragged by, everyone was longing for nightfall. At the Lion Brewery and the Eley detonator works, at Claudius Ash's Mineral Tooth Manufactory and Nichol's Waterproofing and Cloth Pressing plant, and at Mr Holmes's great slaughterhouse on the corner of Marshall Street, the workers waited restlessly for the day's work finally to be over so they could make their way home. In the schools and the shops, the dining houses and the pubs and the great parish workhouse on Poland Street, they sweated and grumbled, but when darkness finally came, far from bringing relief, the atmosphere was more oppressive than ever.

Indoors it was stifling, and people coming back from work hurried to throw open their windows, but the air that rolled in on clouds of dust from the street was even hotter and fouler than that in their stuffy little rooms, and they were forced out again. Small groups stood around their front doors, vainly trying to get a breath of air. Dr Clarke, one of Rogers's colleagues, was in Broad Street that day and knew the place well. He told a meeting of the Westminster Medical Society that he had never known the atmosphere so bad as on that Thursday night. The air in Soho was scarcely respirable, he said.

Even so, no one could have predicted what was to come. Late that night and into the early hours of the following morning, 200 people in that tiny patch of west Soho – a cluster of lanes and alleys of little more than 400 by 200 yards – were simultaneously struck down without warning by an explosion of cholera more swift and deadly than has ever been seen in Britain before or since. There were none of the usual symptoms, not even a few hours of diarrhoea. People who at one moment seemed full of life collapsed in agony, and within hours they were dead. The disease swept through the streets like an act of biblical vengeance, respecting neither physical strength nor social position, and outdoing notorious outbreaks like Albion Terrace and Drouet's Asylum with its virulence and speed of attack.

Whole families were carried off together or, even worse, reduced to one sole survivor, and children who had gone to sleep with two parents woke up to find themselves orphans. The victims included young men at the peak of fitness as well as frail old women and those already half-dead from other illnesses, and the better-off classes in the private houses of Great Pulteney Street died just as surely as the Irish immigrants in the Peter Street tenements. Cholera killed milkmen and milliners, publicans and policemen, cabinetmakers and coffee-house workers and, most of all, the tailors and their wives and children, who earnt their living supplying the fashionable outfitters of nearby Regent Street and Bond Street, and who made up most of the residents of the Broad Street area.

Before daybreak the next morning those who were still able to stand were out on the streets, panic-stricken and running in all directions, desperately trying to get help, but there was little to be had. Local doctors like Rogers and Clarke were run off their feet, and most of the victims were dead long before a medical man could reach them. The clergy hurried from house to house, bringing what comfort they could to the dying and the bereaved while they themselves were in a state of shock. By noon, hysteria had already begun to give way to stunned silence and grief. People gathered in the lanes, huddled together, white-faced and terrified. Women stood weeping in the road, and children wandered about dazed, with no one left to look after them.

And so it continued over that weekend and throughout the following week. On Sunday, 127 died, and on the Monday, seventy-six. Ten days later, the death toll stood at an astounding 500 and still rising. Proportionately, it was as devastating as anything that, centuries earlier, the plague had ever delivered. The records make hard reading. At number 1 Berwick Street, six people were struck down and five of them died. A few doors away, in the rooms over Timson's grocers shop, seven died. In St Ann's Court and St Ann's Place, where many of the poorest families lived, forty-six lost their lives, including a woman whose five relatives had to sleep in the same room as her corpse, such was the overcrowding in Soho and the numbers of dead bodies piling up all around.

Three women lived at number 1 Carnaby Street: the mistress of the house, who was twenty-seven; her sister, aged twenty; and their lodger, a forty-year-old housekeeper. Compared with the miserable inhabitants of St Ann's Place, these women were comfortably off, yet over the course of four days all three of them died. A charlady in nearby Silver Street, who shared her humble room with seventeen assorted dogs, cats and rabbits, lost her life, as did two workmen at Claudius Ash's Mineral Tooth Manufactory and three people at the bookbinders in Noel Street, including the master bookbinder and his twenty-three-year-old nephew. Two of the bookbinder workers also went down with the disease but fortunately they recovered, although they were left traumatised by their experiences.

In Hopkins Street, the toll was fifteen deaths; in Cambridge Street, sixteen; in Kemp's Court, nine; in Pulteney Court, twenty-four; in New Street, ten; and there were similar stories in Cross Street, Berwick Street, Marlborough Row, and up and down all the surrounding lanes and alleys. But nothing could compare with Broad Street. The list of victims there has a horrible monotony: six deaths at number 3, four at number 4, three at number 5, one at number 6, two at number 7, seven at no 9, and so on, house by house all the way down both sides of the road. The two deaths at number 7 were of a mother and daughter, both upholsterers by trade; the mother was taken ill at her work and the daughter on her way home from her mother's funeral.

At number 40 Broad Street where the Lewises lived, the story was as dreadful as anywhere. It was here that the little Lewis baby had died of exhaustion and diarrhoea just thirty-six hours after the outbreak began. Two hours after the child's death, one of the Lewises' fellow tenants, a twenty-five-year-old tailor, died of cholera in his first-floor back room. His wife followed him on the Tuesday morning. The tenant in the third-floor back, another tailor, lingered long enough to be taken to hospital before he finally succumbed two weeks later. A second woman also died on the third floor, although local opinion was divided about how she met her end: some of the neighbours insisted that she died of fright rather than cholera, and as no medical help could be found for her in time, the matter was left undecided. There was no such ambiguity about the death of baby Lewis's father, however. Forty-six-year-old Police Constable Thomas Lewis went down with cholera on 8 September, a week after his little daughter had passed away, and he died on the 19th. Sarah was left on her own to bring up her remaining two children.

The nearby Middlesex Hospital took most of the cases that managed to make it as far as a hospital, and its doctors fought a valiant battle. The final death rate at the Middlesex was fifty-three per cent – much lower than that estimated on the streets – although those who survived long enough to be admitted probably had a higher-than-average natural chance of recovery. Even so, the orderlies were trundling the bodies to the mortuary as fast as they were carrying new patients on to the wards. During the first three days of the outbreak, the head physician, Septimus Sibley, admitted 120 cases and sent many more over to University College Hospital. At the same time Mr Sibley issued an urgent appeal for more staff, and among those reporting for duty was the superintendent of a London nursing home, a dedicated and determined woman called Florence Nightingale.

That summer, thirty-three-year-old Florence had taken up her first hospital post after battling for years with her family and friends to be allowed to do something more useful than arranging flowers and attending balls. Nursing was regarded with particular horror by polite society, not only for the distressing and unseemly nature of the work, but also because nurses had a reputation for drunkenness and promiscuity. Nevertheless in 1854, Miss Nightingale found herself running a charitable establishment, the Institution for the Care of Sick Gentlewomen, at number 1 Harley Street. The clinic had just been opened by some of Florence's aristocratic friends, and she persuaded them to give her a job, overcoming their misgivings about employing a woman from their own background in such an unsuitable role. Even so, despite her pleasure in making a start in her chosen occupation, Florence described her new place of work rather condescendingly as 'a sanatorium for sick governesses run by a committee of fine ladies'.

It was not surprising then that when the Middlesex sent out its SOS, Florence Nightingale at once volunteered for what would surely prove to be the challenge she craved. She was not disappointed. Her friend, the writer Elizabeth Gaskell, told how at the height of the crisis the hospital was admitting patients from the Broad Street area every half an hour, and how Florence stayed up day and night, undressing them as they arrived and applying turpentine fomentations. 'All through the night the wretched, shrieking creatures were being carried in . . . she was never off her feet,' Mrs Gaskell wrote.

According to Florence, one particular underclass was especially badly hit. 'The prostitutes came in perpetually, poor creatures, staggering off their beat. It took worse hold of them than of any,' Gaskell reported. However, no other contemporary accounts mention this, and the idea may well owe something to Nightingale's sanctimonious views about 'fallen women'. At least one of Florence's stories seems to have acquired a measure of Victorian piety in the telling: 'One poor girl, loathsomely filthy, came in and was dead in four hours,' Nightingale said. 'I held her in my arms and I heard her saying something. I bent down to hear: "Pray God that you may never be in the despair I am in at this time."'

Nightingale and a porter were the only hospital staff on duty that night, according to Mrs Gaskell. All the other nurses had collapsed with exhaustion, Gaskell said, and although some medical students came in smoking cigars, they went away again as another prostitute was carried in: 'FN undressed the woman, who was half tipsy but kept saying: "You would not think it ma'am, but a week ago I was in silk and satins, dancing at Woolwich."' As if to endorse the views of Miss Nightingale's family about her choice of career, the woman in question had been supplementing her income from prostitution with a little part-time nursing.

Less than two months later, Florence Nightingale left England with a hand-picked team of nurses bound for Scutari and the sick and wounded of the Crimea. There she was to fight filthy hospitals, poor supplies, incompetent officials, infected wounds, dysentery and, of course, cholera, with equal ferocity. In the process she lay the foundations of the modern nursing profession.

While the Middlesex was the nearest conventional hospital to Broad Street, another medical establishment found itself right in the centre of the epidemic. The London Homeopathic Hospital, with just twenty-five beds, was on Golden Square, a minute's walk from Broad Street. It had been opened five years earlier by Dr Frederick Foster Hervey Quin, a colourful character who was a close friend of Charles Dickens and physician to Queen Victoria's uncle, Prince Leopold. Quin had studied on the Continent with

Samuel Hahnemann, the founder of homeopathy, and saw it as his mission to bring this unusual new therapy to the common people. Homeopathy then, as now, was regarded by many with suspicion and even contempt. Its guiding principle of treating like with like – prescribing small doses of remedies that themselves cause the symptoms of the illness in order to prompt the body's natural defences into action – is not the problem for conventional medical science. This, after all, is the principle upon which vaccination is founded. The real difficulty for orthodox medicine is homeopathy's method of diluting its remedies to such an extent that not one molecule of the active ingredient remains in the medicine that is given to the patient. The arguments continue today about whether water has a 'memory' and is capable of retaining the characteristics of other substances long after they have been diluted out of existence.

In 1849, as the London Homeopathic was preparing to open its doors, a Parisian hospital handed over some of its beds to a group of homeopathic practitioners, hoping that they might have some success where conventional cholera treatments had failed. The homeopaths set to work with some of their standard *materia medica* such as bryony, charcoal and, in particular, arsenic. Cholera's symptoms are not unlike those of acute arsenic poisoning – copious diarrhoea, vomiting, cold clammy skin, a fast drop in body temperature, convulsions and coma, with death following in a few hours – and so, according to homeopathy's principle of treating like with like, a minute dose of the poison would seem to be indicated. There is, however, one major drawback in using arsenic in the treatment of cholera: it doesn't work, any more than any of the then standard treatments worked, and all seven of the French patients died. 'These facts will be a warning to those who would be inclined to give faith to the magnificent promises of homeopathists,' pronounced the *Lancet* smugly.

And that same year, a London inquest jury under deputy-coroner Henry Wakley, son of the *Lancet* editor Thomas Wakley, who as a coroner himself presided over the Drouet hearings, returned a verdict of manslaughter on a self-taught homeopath called Charles

Pearce. Pearce was accused of having starved his brother to death while attempting to cure him of cholera, and was hauled off to Newgate prison after Wakley junior delivered a damning summing up of the evidence, including some pointed remarks on the subject of quackery. Hahnemann himself recommended treating cholera patients with camphor for reasons that are not entirely clear. In toxic doses, camphor does produce some cholera-like symptoms such as nausea, vomiting, colic, rigidity and muscle spasms, but its other effects – for example, a high temperature and fast pulse – are quite dissimilar.

In the Soho epidemic, however, homeopathy appeared to chalk up a remarkable success: the London Homeopathic Hospital's mortality rate was just sixteen per cent compared with the Middlesex's fifty-three per cent – which was in line with the general average death rate from cholera at the time – and there was a row when the president of the Royal College of Physicians deliberately omitted this statistic from a report to Parliament. In the light of current knowledge, it is clear that in the treatment of cholera at least, homeopathy has nothing to offer, but in the nineteenth century homeopathy's disdain for procedures like blood-letting meant that its practitioners tended to do less harm than their more orthodox colleagues. It may well be that the higher recovery rates at the London Homeopathic Hospital were due not so much to the homeopaths' ability to cure their patients, but rather to the tendency of the doctors at the Middlesex to kill theirs.

As the cases in Soho during that first week continued to spiral out of control, it wasn't only the hospitals and local doctors who were struggling to cope. The undertakers too were having great difficulties in keeping up with their workload and soon the familiar rumours started to spread that decency was being cast aside in the panic to dispose of the corpses. Certainly many of the victims went to that most ignominious end, a pauper's grave; the parish paid out for over 200 such funerals, many of them not because the deceased couldn't afford the cost of their own burial but because their friends and relatives who would normally have seen to the arrangements were themselves dead or dying. People reported seeing piles of bodies being bundled out of houses and driven away wholesale in carts because there weren't enough hearses to go round, and a deputation from Dufour's Place off Broad Street went to Whitehall to complain about the makeshift mortuary that had been set up in their street.

The death toll would have been higher still but for the numbers who fled the district. Six days after the outbreak began, more than three-quarters of those in the worst-affected streets had packed up what they could and left town. The poorer people with few possessions to worry about were the first to go, but immediately after came their more affluent neighbours, now with more important worries than the safety of their worldly goods.

But flight, of course, was no guarantee of escape, as five years earlier the Reverend Thomas Harrison of Albion Terrace had discovered. One family left their home in Bentinck Street on the morning of Monday, 4 September, for the safety of a relative's house in Gravesend, having watched the drama unfold over the weekend. After all, there were not only their existing children to think of, there was a new baby expected in four weeks and at Gravesend they would be able to breathe more easily. But at seven o'clock the next morning, a few hours after arriving in Kent, the pregnant woman collapsed and two of her children with her. The children recovered but their mother was not so lucky. She finally died on 15 September after managing, somehow, to give birth to her baby.

Then, ten days after it struck and as mysteriously as it had appeared, the epidemic appeared to be over. By 14 September both the daily death toll and the numbers of newly diagnosed fatal cases were down to single figures, and on 30 September, exactly one month after that first night, both deaths and new cases hit zero. The immediate shock and panic were over. Soho could take down the sober government posters listing the measures recommended for containing the disease. It could withdraw the parish leaflets advising those left destitute by the death of a breadwinner how to apply for assistance. It could wash the last of the milky, disinfectant

lime from its cobblestones and contemplate trying to resume something akin to a normal daily life. But as the shops re-opened and
the fugitives drifted back to their homes, hard questions began to
be asked. Why here? Why now?

And there was something else. Even before the last corpse was
hurried off the scene it had become clear that, virulent as it was, the
outbreak had stayed extraordinarily local. All the victims, including the lucky few who recovered, lived or worked within just 250
yards of the corner of Cambridge Street and Broad Street, north of
Golden Square – all, that was, except for a handful of people inex-
plicably singled out for misfortune.

Susannah Eley was the fifty-nine-year-old widow of William
Eley, whose family firm made percussion caps, or detonators, and
employed 200 workmen at its premises on Broad Street. The business flourished in the hands of the Eley's sons, and the company
was to become so well known that forty years later Sir Arthur
Conan Doyle had Sherlock Holmes refer to it in a story called
'The Speckled Band': 'And so Watson, if you are ready, we shall
call a cab and drive to Waterloo. I should be very much obliged if
you would slip your revolver into your pocket. An Eley's No. 2 is
an excellent argument with gentlemen who can twist steel pokers
into knots. That and a tooth-brush are, I think, all that we need.'
In fact, Conan Doyle was confusing Eley, the cartridge-makers,
with Webley, the gunsmiths, but he knew that his readers would
instantly recognise the name.

Back in the 1850s, the Eleys were already successful enough for
Susannah to move from the family's lodgings above the noisy, polluted Broad Street factory to the green open spaces of West
Hampstead, and by the summer of 1854, Susannah hadn't set foot
in Soho for months. On Friday, 1 September – at exactly the same
time that the epidemic struck Broad Street – Susannah Eley was
taken violently ill with cholera, the only case in the whole of
Hampstead. She died the next day. Susannah's niece from Islington
who was staying with her aunt spent another night in Hampstead
before making her way home. Hardly had she arrived back in

Islington, however, when she too collapsed and died. And like Susannah, the niece was the only case of cholera in her entire neighbourhood. Yet Susannah's sons who, after all, worked in the middle of Broad Street, stayed perfectly healthy through the entire outbreak – which was even odder considering that eighteen of their workers died.

Unlike Mrs Eley, Mr Wickwar was already in poor health, but when he heard that his brother John was seriously ill in Soho he left Brighton at once for London. Still, he was too late. By the time he reached the house in Poland Street, John was dead, just twelve hours after being struck down. Mr Wickwar decided against seeing the body. Perhaps he wanted to remember his brother alive and healthy, rather than as a corpse bearing all the signs of a horrible disease. Perhaps he was simply frightened. Whatever his reasons, he was in the house for only twenty minutes; just long enough to throw down a few mouthfuls of steak and a small glass of brandy and water before setting off once again, this time for Pentonville in north London where he was spending the night. Yet despite his hurry, he couldn't escape the taint of Soho. That evening Mr Wickwar was seized by cholera and by morning he, like his brother John, was dead.

Another particularly unfortunate victim was an army officer from St John's Wood who came to Wardour Street merely to dine on that Thursday evening. The Soho supper was his last.

But just as these three were especially unlucky, so other people enjoyed an escape that seemed nothing short of miraculous. The epidemic was mainly concentrated in two blocks bounded by Broad Street, Silver Street, New Street and Marshall Street. Henry Whitehead, the young curate of St Luke's in Berwick Street, worked out that if you started from the western end of Broad Street and walked down the south side to the eastern end, walked back as far as the brewery and then along Hopkins Street, Husband Street, New Street and Pulteney Court, you would pass forty-five houses on your way, only six of which had escaped without a death. In fact, the situation was even worse: Whitehead was only thinking about the residents. The Eley percussion cap factory took up two of those houses and eighteen of its workers died, uncounted, in their homes in other parts of London.

The next block down, bounded by Berwick Street, was also badly affected but for a curious exception. Not one of the work-men from the Lion Brewery nor any of the clergy or lay workers from Whitehead's church, right in the centre of the outbreak, fell sick. Yet seven builders working on a site next door to the brewery were taken ill in one day, and in a little block of four houses just fif-teen yards from St Luke's, thirty-two people died. The Poland Street workhouse was another case that defied explanation. Out of 535 inmates, there were only five deaths, although many of the sick were brought in to be cared for in the infirmary and died on the premises.

The final death toll of the 1854 Broad Street outbreak was cer-tainly over 600, but how much over no one can say. Like the mother from Bentinck Street, some people fled the district only to die elsewhere from the disease they had carried with them, while others perished unrecorded in a hospital or workhouse, and yet more, like the labourers at the Eley percussion cap factory, died in their homes in a different part of London. The true scale of the tragedy will never be known.

On the evening of 7 September, a week into the outbreak and with the death count at 458 and rising, the local Board of Guardians met at their customary venue, the vestry hall next to St James's Church in Piccadilly. As guardians, they bore much of the respon-sibility for public health and safety in the parish of St James's Westminster, but no one could accuse them of being over zealous in the way that they were currently discharging their duties. As soon as the government had heard about the tragedy, it sent a medical officer over to Soho to advise the guardians as they supposedly set about their tasks of disinfecting streets and houses and making suitable arrangements for the sick and dying, but when Mr Patterson arrived on the scene he discovered that there was little happening for him to advise on. He reported back to Whitehall that he had found the parish 'in the very midst of a frightful outbreak' and was astounded by their lack of action.

Now as the sombre band of local worthies contemplated the chaos before them and pondered helplessly on what to do, a stranger turned up at the vestry hall and asked politely for permission to speak. He had something to say about the cholera. The board was not in the habit of granting audiences to anyone who happened to wander in off the streets, and it was hard to imagine that this odd, shy, insignificant-looking man could possibly have anything useful to contribute, but these were, after all, strange times, and the board decided that they might as well hear him out.

After all, it wasn't as though anyone else had much to suggest.

CHAPTER 12

The Big Idea

In a case in which lives may depend upon steps being taken scientif-ically and promptly, all delicacies to the caprices and prejudices of a few leading men ought to be cast aside

Home Secretary Lord Palmerston to Sir Benjamin Hall, President of the Board of Health, August 1854

While the St James's Board of Guardians were collectively wringing their hands in Piccadilly, half a mile or so away over in Whitehall Sir Benjamin Hall, 1st Baronet Llanover, had been busy. On 12 August, just two weeks before the Broad Street epidemic struck, and with the country now in the grip of its third cholera epidemic, the rumbustious Lord Palmerston, who was now the Home Secretary, had appointed Sir Benjamin to replace Edwin Chadwick at the Board of Health. As Foreign Secretary in 1831, Palmerston had been concerned with tracking the disease as it moved across the Continent, but his responsibilities were now for internal affairs and in nineteenth-century Britain that included the health of the nation.

Shortly before Hall got his feet under his new desk, his prede-cessor at the Board, the deeply unpopular Chadwick, had been subjected to a scathing attack in the House of Commons, not least from Hall himself. In a long speech, Sir Benjamin did a step-by-step demolition job on Chadwick's entire personality and career, accusing him of ignorance, incompetence and opportunism at every turn, and quoting one of the Poor Law commissioners who had dubbed him 'an unscrupulous and dangerous man'. Back in the 1830s when, as secretary to the Poor Law Commission, Chadwick was responsible for the workhouses, he introduced rules of such 'atrocious stringency', separating men from their wives and parents from their children, that the law itself was thrown into disrepute, Hall claimed, and while for the past twenty years Chadwick had held a whole series of important and mostly well-paid jobs, the practical service that he had rendered to the community remained to be discovered.

The Parliamentary knives were clearly out for Chadwick. A few days after Hall's comprehensive character assassination, Lord Seymour weighed in. The Board of Health's advice was worse than useless, he told MPs, while the cost of publishing it was frightful; Chadwick was currently spending over £250,000 a year on disseminating his prejudiced, one-sided documents. No fewer than 6,000 copies of the 'Report on Extramural Sepulture' [siting burial grounds away from built-up areas] had been printed, for example, 'a lengthy document of no practical use to the general community, but pleasing to the Board as an advertisement of their own merits,' said Seymour.

The government had finally had enough of this troublesome bureaucrat who had proved a little too opinionated and zealous for many people's liking, alienating the medical profession with his lack of regard for its sensibilities and upsetting property owners and water companies with his vociferous demands for reform. Having lost the confidence of Parliament in such a spectacular fashion, Edwin Chadwick and his friends had no option but to resign, and Palmerston was now determined to have an MP in the job, someone who understood the political niceties and who could be easily reined in if he showed any signs of following in Chadwick's uncompromising footsteps.

Sir Benjamin Hall was the Member for the London constituency of Marylebone; a tall, imposing and – despite his attack on

Chadwick – usually amiable man, who was known to his colleagues as Big Ben. Hall was later to be responsible for overseeing the building of the gothic fantasy that is Britain's Houses of Parliament, and his fellow MPs, in a cheerful mood, took his nickname and gave it to the massive new bell on the St Stephen's clock tower. An aristocrat whose family owned extensive lands in south Wales, his marriage to another member of the gentry, Augusta Waddington, had united the two great estates of Abercarn and Llanover in the principality.

Enthusiastic patrons of Welsh culture, the couple were great promoters of the country's history and language, in Augusta's case to the point of obsession. Lady Llanover, who called herself Gwenynen Gwent – the Honey Bee of Gwent – distinguished herself by inventing what is now regarded as the Welsh national costume, complete with shawl and tall conical hat. A fervent teetotaller, another of her claims to fame was to buy up all the pubs in the area, give them Welsh names and turn them into tea shops. Locally, the couple were probably regarded as something of a mixed blessing.

The August of 1854, however, found Sir Benjamin in London with rather more pressing matters on his mind than clock towers or *eisteddfodau* and, despite a usually leisurely manner, he moved fast to tackle the task before him. One of his first actions in the face of this latest cholera attack was to appoint medical inspectors to draft some hygiene regulations and to try to press the parish authorities into clearing away filth and disinfecting the streets. Dealing with the parishes was no mean job, however, as others had found before him, and Hall was greatly hampered by the absolute chaos that was local government, and his own lack of authority over it. A plethora of committees, boards and bodies responsible for different aspects of local health jostled for position and power in town and country parishes all over Britain, and London was a particular bureaucratic nightmare.

Local government was largely in the hands of the parishes, whose main tier consisted of a Board of Guardians and a Vestry committee, but alongside the guardians and the Vestry came the highways boards, the paving commissioners, the sewers commissioners, the improvement commissioners, the water companies, the gas companies, the police and the magistrates, all of whom had a finger in the pie. Hall had to deal in the main with the boards of guardians, some of whom, five years earlier, had failed so badly in their duty of care to their young charges at Drouet's establishment in Tooting. The guardians were concerned with the plight of the poor as well as with many aspects of public health and safety. They also suggested the rate of local taxation needed to look after the destitute, but the financial clout lay with the vestries, which had to approve expenditure.

Just days after Hall assumed his duties, he found himself involved in a row in Harwich where the guardians were refusing to allow the body of a sailor who had died of cholera to be brought ashore. The Harwich authorities thought it a much better plan for the ship to continue on to Hull and unload its problem there instead. In the meantime, the unfortunate man lay buried in the ship's cargo of chalk while the argument raged on. Hall was disgusted. He telegraphed the guardians that the body should be brought ashore immediately and given 'a proper and Christian burial'. A Board of Health order to that effect bearing his signature would be in the next post.

Ironically before he took charge at the Board, Hall had been a great champion of the rights of the parishes to manage their own affairs and he loathed Chadwick's authoritarian views about centralised control, but the difficulties now confronting him quickly made him change his mind. He was soon telling Palmerston: 'The first and most obvious necessity in the metropolis is to sweep away the existing chaos of local jurisdictions and to constitute local boards of health ... with ample powers to deal with the evils.' Until that could be done, however, he was stuck with the situation and – egged on by the ebullient Home Secretary – he wrote to every board of guardians offering government assistance. If they accepted, a medical officer was sent. If they rejected his help, Hall decided to demand a full report of their current situation regarding cholera and the measures they were taking. Where areas were particularly badly hit, inspectors would make house-to-house calls.

This was still not enough for the no-nonsense Palmerston once he too realised the nature of the problem. In London where the disease now had a real hold, Hall should just send a medical officer to any district where cholera was reported with no further ado, the Home Secretary thought. The matter was too urgent for niceties, and waiting around for ignorant and self-important parishmen to decide whether to accept help was wasting precious time. Hundreds of lives should not have to depend on the whims of a few local dignitaries. And besides, people would often take advice if it were given them on the spot, even if they had originally refused it, Palmerston believed. The English tradesman – by which he meant the typical local ratepayer and also the typical local vestryman – had many good qualities, the Home Secretary told his junior minister, but he harboured an exaggerated idea of his own wisdom and he would do anything to avoid a rate rise. In fact, he was often prepared to see his neighbours die around him and risk his own life and that of his wife and children rather than try to ward off the danger if so doing would mean sixpence on the rates. Hall took the point, and by 4 September his inspectors were at work both north and south of the Thames.

But even as Sir Benjamin began introducing the anti-cholera measures that previous governments had urged with such notable lack of success, and as he plotted with the Home Secretary to force the parishes to clean up their act, Hall had decided that something much more radical was called for. They were all still scratching around in the dark. It didn't take a member of the Royal College of Physicians to see that there was some link between cholera and bad living conditions, but what exactly was it? Why was this terrible Asian scourge, unknown in Britain twenty-five years before, now breaking out with dreadful regularity all over the country? How was it being spread? Why did it decimate some towns and villages but leave others alone? And what made it stop so suddenly in one area, only to reappear without warning elsewhere?

Pondering the matter as thousands had done so before him, Hall came up with a visionary plan. He would bring together a team of the country's leading doctors and scientists to look into every conceivable aspect of this disease. The work would be on a far grander scale than anything previously attempted, and the more he thought about it, the more he felt convinced that such a comprehensive study would provide the answers. Back in 1830, the Russians had offered a £50,000 prize for the best treatise on cholera, but Hall's project was to be designed, funded and controlled directly by the state. It would be the first time that a British government had ever set up a scientific inquiry and paid for it out of the public purse.

Hall outlined his thinking to his new boss:

The object will be to institute in the metropolis, both in infected and uninfected districts, enquiries and observations as to air and water, both microscopic, meteorological and chemical, and to put a complete return from all medical practitioners of all cases treated by them, under forms prepared here, so as to elect a greater body of information on the medical part of the question than has yet been got together.

With Palmerston's blessing, on 24 August, just a week before the Broad Street outbreak and while a solitary John Snow was tramping the streets of south London collecting information about water supplies for his 'Grand Experiment', Hall summoned two leaders of the medical profession, John Ayrton Paris, president of the Royal College of Physicians, and William Lawrence, surgeon to Queen Victoria and vice-president of the Royal College of Surgeons, to his office in Whitehall to hear his plans. A politician to the core, Hall knew that the co-operation of these powerful men was essential if his inquiry were to stand any chance of success. It was a very different approach from that of the abrasive Chadwick who had managed to upset the entire medical establishment almost to a man, and even the *Lancet* was quick to welcome this new climate of co-operation and respect between politics and medicine:

'Nothing probably more powerfully contributed to the downfall of the late board than the want of consideration evidenced towards the medical profession. Sir Benjamin is possessed of known ability and has a thorough knowledge of business; moreover, although not wanting in firmness, he is of a conciliatory disposition.'

Ayrton Paris and Lawrence listened carefully as Hall explained his big idea and then they quickly assured him that he could count on the support of the doctors. There was of course the small matter of fees to be arranged, however. Two guineas per man per day would not be unreasonable, they thought. Hall did some fast calculations and put the likely bill at £200 for the year. Quite a bargain, he told himself. Quickly, he drew his team together. The main investigation he put in the hands of five men, who together would comprise what was known as the Committee for Scientific Inquiry. One was William Farr from the Registrar General's office, who had left medicine to become a compiler of abstracts; in other words, a statistician. It was Farr's breakdowns of cholera deaths that John Snow was currently using to identify which doors to knock upon in south London.

With Farr would be William Baly, assistant physician to St Bartholomew's Hospital and to the Millbank Penitentiary. Baly had dismissed John Snow's ideas the previous year in a report he wrote with William Gull for the Royal College of Physicians. The pair had also delivered the College's damning verdict on Budd, Swayne and Brittan five years earlier, when the Bristol doctors had claimed to have discovered the cause of the disease. The other members of Hall's committee were John Simon, surgeon to St Thomas's Hospital and medical officer for the City of London; Richard Owen, professor of zoology at the Royal College of Surgeons; and Neil Arnott, physician extraordinary to Queen Victoria, who had worked with Edwin Chadwick on his report into the living conditions of the poor. To advise on treatment were illustrious names such as Ayrton Paris himself, and Nathaniel Ward, master of the Society of Apothecaries, the body that had proved so intractable when John Snow asked to sit his exams three months early.

Some aspects of the research – for example, the effects of the disease on the body and its treatment – had of course been vigorously debated for over thirty-five years, but Hall was determined that this exercise would be comprehensive, pulling all of the strands together and examining the evidence in a truly scientific manner. The study of the water and the atmosphere was quite new, he believed, and he was excited at the prospect of the groundbreaking information that might emerge once his experts set to work. Clearly none of the members of the Committee for Scientific Inquiry thought it worth telling their new boss about the ideas of John Snow, who at the time was engaged in the most methodical investigation into the relationship between cholera and the water supply that anyone, certainly including the British government, would devise. While the committee almost certainly knew nothing of Snow's current research in south London, William Baly at least was familiar with the theory that cholera was largely water-borne and spread through the oral-fecal route, even though he didn't believe it. Baly, with William Gull, had after all discussed Snow's ideas in a report for the Royal College of Physicians the previous year, although only to pronounce them 'untenable'.

For the microscopical, meteorological and chemical work, Sir Benjamin recruited Arthur Hill Hassall from London's Royal Free Hospital; James Glaisher, superintendent of the magnetic and meteorological department at the Royal Observatory at Greenwich; and Robert Thomson, lecturer in chemistry at St Thomas's Hospital.

Arthur Hill Hassall was a contemporary of John Snow and had studied medicine in Dublin. As well as practising day to day as a busy doctor in London, including a stint in the then appalling slums of Notting Hill, Hassall was an experienced microscopist and chemist with interests ranging right across the spectrum of the natural sciences. He published works on anatomy and physiology, chemistry, pathology, botany and zoology, but in particular on hygiene and public health. When Hall recruited him for the Committee for Scientific Inquiry, Hassall had already published a booklet on the contamination and the living creatures in London's water, but he was more famous for his collaboration with Thomas Wakley of the *Lancet*.

As he went about his business on the streets of the capital, Hassall had noticed the many dubious-looking items of food on display in shop windows and the extravagant claims made for them by the shopkeepers. He was particularly struck by the doubtful quality of much of the coffee on sale, so he bought samples of roasted coffee from several different shops and subjected them to a close microscopical and chemical examination. Hardly any turned out to be pure coffee. Some consisted almost entirely of chicory, while others contained large amounts of roasted wheat, rye, beans, peas or burnt sugar. 'These spurious admixtures were sold under the most grandiloquent of names with statements that were absolutely false,' Hassall said.

Having damned the coffee trade, Hassall next turned his attention to brown sugar. There was already considerable popular suspicion about this product, as shown by the often repeated but possibly apocryphal story of the grocer who was said to have summoned his assistant up from the cellar with the words: 'Have you watered the treacle and sanded the sugar?' 'Yes.' 'Then come up to prayers.' While Hassall found little evidence of sand in his sugar samples, he found something just as unpleasant: 'Most of the brown sugar . . . abounded with living and dead louse-like creatures in all stages of growth and development, from the ova upwards to the perfect parasite.' The louse-like creature was in fact the *Tyrogluphus sacchari*, or sugar mite, responsible, as Hassall realised, for the then common skin irritation known as grocer's itch.

This was the type of investigation precisely calculated to appeal to the campaigning Thomas Wakley, doctor, coroner, MP and editor of the *Lancet*, who could never leave a possible scandal unprobed. Wakley contacted Hassall to congratulate him but told him that, admirable as his work was, he would never do any lasting good until he was able to tell the public exactly where he had bought his samples. 'Do you think it would be possible to do this without an amount of risk that might be ruinous?' Wakley asked Hassall. 'I replied yes, I believed it might be done,' Hassall recalled.

The result was a Victorian exercise in consumer rights: a regular series of investigative articles on different types of food and drink, as well as drugs, tobacco and snuff, published in the *Lancet* during the early 1850s under the grand title 'Reports of the Analytical Sanitary Commission' and complete with detailed illustrations of the microscopic findings, as well as the names and addresses of the suppliers concerned. In fact, the impressive-sounding Analytical Sanitary Commission consisted solely of Hassall and his illustrator Mr Miller, who would sally out at night in all weathers on their shopping expeditions equipped with paper bags, labels and ink for their samples. 'These nocturnal excursions brought us into many curious parts of London and gave us a wonderful insight into the habits and ways of life of people in the poor districts,' Hassall said.

Their revelations caused a public outcry. There was scarcely an item of food or drink on sale anywhere in London, or so it seemed, that had not been diluted with water, bulked out with inferior ingredients or mixed with unpleasant and sometimes dangerous chemicals to strengthen the colour or flavour. Much of the milk tested consisted largely of water. Nearly every loaf contained huge quantities of alum (a chemical compound, potassium aluminum phosphate), which improved the appearance and the texture of bread baked with poor quality flour. Cayenne pepper contained sawdust, large amounts of 'ferruginous earth, resembling brick dust' as well as the metal, red lead. Hardly any of the vinegar samples were what they purported to be. Royal Standard vinegar, for example, advertised as being 'manufactured entirely from malt and highly recommended for its purity and strength' was found to be manufactured entirely from a small amount of malt and a huge amount of sulphuric acid. There were marmalades and jams consisting largely of turnips; cocoa composed mainly of flour, corn meal and tapioca; tea containing china clay, rice and a chemical dye known as Prussian blue; and porter to which strychnine and vitriol had been added. Fortnum and Mason, no less, were caught selling anchovies in a brine vinegar that had been dyed with a large helping of red earth, as well as a greengage jam whose 'deep and unnatural' hue owed its brilliance not to fruit but to copper. Crosse and Blackwell of Soho Square were caught out in a similar seafood scam – namely passing off cheap, coarse fish as anchovies with the help of coloured clay.

Altogether over the course of four years, Hassall reported on over 2,500 different samples, and the resulting scandal over his findings forced the government to bring in new laws on food adulteration. And while Wakley received a barrage of furious letters from shopkeepers and their lawyers, Hassall's diligence and accuracy ensured that not one of them ever resulted in a court case.

John Snow was later to become interested in food adulteration – in his case in its effects on health – and in 1857 he published a paper arguing that there was a link between the bread additive, alum and the bone deformity, rickets, which develops in childhood. Rickets was then widespread among working-class Londoners, but rare in the equally deprived parts of Yorkshire and Northumbria that Snow knew well. He believed that this was because people in the villages ate home-baked, alum-free bread. We now know that lack of exposure to sunlight at least partly explains why London children were more at risk from the disease than their country counterparts, but doctors in the mid-nineteenth century already understood that rickets is a deficiency disease caused by a lack of calcium phosphate in the bones. Snow's argument was that continual large doses of alum interfered with the body's ability to absorb calcium phosphate from the diet. The theory remains unproven, but other aluminum salts have been shown to interfere with phosphate absorption even, occasionally, to the extent of causing rickets.

The meteorologist member of Hall's team, James Glaisher of the Royal Observatory, placed his faith firmly in his own branch of science to come up with the required answers. Convinced that the weather held the key not only to cholera, but to many of the epidemic diseases currently plaguing the country, he wrote:

> I have little hesitation in saying that, were the meteorology of our towns carefully ascertained and collated with that of the metropolis, and both together with that of the country generally, that in a short time we should be in a condition to elaborate a clear insight into the meteorological causes of cholera, influenza and many phases of disease which now burst upon us with the suddenness and devastating power of a divine and wrathful visitation.

Glaisher was later to become something of a public hero by taking part in a daring adventure. He and a balloonist called Henry Coxwell embarked on a series of flights in order to collect meteorological data, and on 5 September 1862, they took off from Wolverhampton and reached a recording-breaking height of 30,000 feet without oxygen, nearly dying in the attempt. Glaisher lost consciousness and, on the brink of collapse himself, Coxwell climbed up into the rigging to free a tangled valve line and prevent the balloon from going any higher and killing them both by hypothermia or oxygen starvation. His hands were paralysed with cold but he managed to tug the cord with his teeth.

All had been well until they reached 26,000 feet, Glaisher said, but then as he tried to take another set of altitude and temperature readings:

> I could not see the fine column of the mercury in the tube; then the fine divisions on the scale of the instrument became invisible ... Shortly afterwards I laid my arm upon the table, possessed of its full vigour; but directly after, being desirous of using it, I found it powerless ... I then tried to move the other arm, but found it powerless also ... I seemed to have no legs ... My head fell on my left shoulder. I struggled, and shook my body, but could not move my arms. I got my head upright, but for an instant only, when it fell on my right shoul-

der; and then I fell backwards . . . I dimly saw Mr Coxwell, and
endeavoured to speak, but could not do so. There was an
instant intense black darkness, and the optic nerve lost power
suddenly. I thought . . . death would come unless we speedily
descended. Other thoughts were actively entering my mind
when I suddenly became unconscious.

When Coxwell finally succeeded in rousing him, Glaisher saw
that his friend's hands had turned black with cold. Extraordinarily,
though, the pair suffered no long-term nor even short-term ill
effects, and when they finally came down in the middle of the
Shropshire countryside, they were able to walk the eight miles to
the nearest inn. 'They penetrated into that distant region of the
skies in which it has been satisfactorily proved that no life can be
long maintained . . . and were so nearly sacrificed to their unselfish
daring,' wrote one admirer.

Hall's new Medical Council met on 6 September, the day before the
St James's parishmen held their less learned deliberations. Before
the Council was a letter from Sir Benjamin explaining that his aim
was to 'deduce from this terrible visitation both facts and lessons
which may hereafter be made available'. He had received support
from many quarters, he told them, 'But the most valuable result
within my reach at the present will be wanting unless I have your
aid in procuring such information upon the concomitants and
course of the epidemic as only medical and scientific observation
can detect.' He clearly had great hopes.

By this time the first reports of the drama unfolding in Broad
Street had reached Whitehall, and consequently on 2 September,
with 200 people dead or dying, Hall had despatched Inspector
Patterson hot-foot over to Soho. Only three weeks into his new
job, the MP was already beginning feel the strain: 'I sit here all day
and direct and order and attend to the many people who call and
most fervently do hope that our exertions may do good and that
ere long we may hear that this sad visitation has abated,' Hall

wrote, adding poignantly: 'The labour of the office is nothing in comparison to the anxiety of mind.'

When Mr Patterson reported back that something quite extraordinary was going on in Broad Street, on a more frightening scale than anything that cholera had ever yet produced in Britain, Hall's response was to order in a hit squad. Three investigators would go from house to house, just as John Snow, unknown and unremarked, was doing in south London; but unlike Snow, who believed he knew exactly what he was looking for, the Board's men were given a huge list of questions to answer. This vicious but highly contained outbreak offered the perfect opportunity to look at cholera's strange behaviour in the greatest possible detail, and Hall was determined to leave no Soho cobblestone unturned.

For each of 800 properties around Broad Street, then, the inspectors had to record the number of occupants: how many of them fell sick; how many died; the occupations of the deceased, their living habits and even the room in which they were taken ill, as well as any other information about the people or their surroundings that the inspectors thought might have some bearing on the matter in hand. The officials also had to report on the physical characteristics of the area; the atmosphere before and during the outbreak; the layout of the streets; the ventilation; the condition of the houses; the smells; the overcrowding; the privies, the drains and the sewers; the general state of cleanliness – and the water supply.

In short, they were to investigate anything and everything that might possibly help to explain why 200 people had been struck down in one night alone and why the local residents had been dying in droves ever since. There had to be something, somewhere, in that little patch of streets that would provide some answers. Accordingly on 5 September, Messrs Fraser, Hughes and Ludlow sharpened their pencils, made their way over to Soho and waded into the misery that was Broad Street.

CHAPTER 13

Proof Positive

On hearing of the late fearful outburst of cholera, the question which we heard asked on all sides is: 'What was the cause?' The very importance of the question makes us diffident in replying to it, nor could we receive any satisfactory answer from the medical practitioners

Board of Health inspectors, Broad Street, 1854

Seven feet below ground, the front basement of number 3 South Row, Soho, was dark, dirty, wet and stinking. It was also home to eight people. When Sir Benjamin Hall's inspectors came to call they commented that the room was a fair specimen of the Soho basements where so many families lived. The back basement at number 3 was occupied by six people, one of whom, Hall's men found, was suffering from what was described as a dangerous attack of choleraic diarrhoea.

South Row was a small alley lined on each side with a brick terrace of narrow, flat-fronted houses, and typical of the dozens of little lanes and pathways that traversed this part of Soho. South Row also resembled the neighbouring streets in that nearly every room in every house was occupied by an entire family. 'As a general consequence,' reported inspectors Fraser, Hughes and Ludlow, 'the passages, stairs and walls are extremely dirty; as well as the interior of the rooms, on entering which we found the air close, oppressive and tainted with a combination of unwholesome odours arising from a number of persons cooking their food, eating, sleeping, washing and drying their clothes in the same apartments, their personal ablutions being little attended to.'

When a group of surgeons visited the basement at number 3 and others like it, again at the request of Sir Benjamin, they voiced their disgust in no uncertain terms: 'We have observed the great number of cellars or underground apartments let out as separate tenements,' they reported. 'We found them generally in a damp and filthy state, with foul smells, without air or ventilation and where no sunshine can penetrate, mere centres of infection and of disease; and we would urge upon the parochial authorities, if they have any regard for the health, decency and comfort of their fellow inhabitants, to have them closed immediately and persons letting out such places prosecuted.'

The problem with that piece of well-meaning advice was that the fellow inhabitants in question had nowhere else to go. For them, the choice was stark: South Row or the streets. Ten days into the epidemic, a reporter visited St Ann's Place at the east end of Broad Street and found the tenants in despair over what they thought was a notice to quit. 'Where can we go to, sir? Although here is not very good, we cannot get better,' they told him. 'Here is the notice but none of us can read, no more can the lady who receives the rent.' In fact, the letter was from the parish ordering the landlord to empty the cesspit and limewash the building within twenty-four hours.

Another journalist making notes near Berwick Street found himself surrounded by a fierce group of Irishmen who assumed he was an official checking up on the overcrowding with a view to getting them evicted. 'The leader, with many angry gesticulations and numerous oaths, said: "I'll have no writing down in my place. Not a divil amongst you shall write anything down here",' the man reported. Reasoning with them was useless, the journalist said, but he understood very well what lay behind the threats: 'Go where you will, you hear complaints as to the difficulty of finding lodgings for "such as they". This is partly the secret of the violence: a shelter for the very poor in London has become so valuable that they suspect us all of endeavouring to rob them of it.'

In the mid-nineteenth century, overcrowding in that part of Soho was just about the worst in the whole of London. On Broad Street alone, where the Lewis family lived, some 860 people were crammed into forty-nine houses, eating, sleeping, washing and defecating, while in nearby Nag's Head Mews, thirty-seven people living in a wooden gallery of small rooms over coach-houses and stables shared a single privy. Sir Benjamin's inspectors found the houses 'almost universally old and inconvenient', and said that with few exceptions – Broad Street, as its name implies, being one – the streets were too narrow for the height of the houses, and the whole place was a claustrophobic maze. The inspectors continued:

> The ends of almost all the streets, instead of being continued by other streets running more or less in line with themselves, cut other streets or turn themselves at right angles and . . . with the exceptions of Golden Square, and the space between Portland Street and Marshall Street, where the workhouse and its grounds stand, there is no open space whatever in the district; the backs of all the streets being filled up with courts, workshops, and warehouses, and here and there with cow-houses and stables. Many of the small streets form culs-de-sac . . . and there is no single street or succession of streets in the whole district down which a free current of air can pass . . . We need hardly add that the ventilation of the district is very bad.

The place had gone downhill fast since it had lost its fashionable status to the up-and-coming Belgravia. The name Soho probably comes from an ancient hunting cry, and Soho Square was laid out in the 1680s on land known as Soho Fields. In the mid-1700s the area was home to the aristocracy but by the beginning of the nine-teenth century the nobility had largely been replaced by the professional classes, the doctors, lawyers and journalists. When they, too, began to drift away the area turned quickly into a slum, its once-fine houses in the hands of absentee landlords and let out by the room.

A friend of the local curate Henry Whitehead described a visit to the priest's patch. First the stranger had to pluck up the courage to dive down one of the many little alleyways off Regent Street:

> Your aim is St Luke's, Berwick Street. You soon see its dim row of dingy, semi-domestic, semi-gothic windows. A man is standing just opposite the barred gate skinning eels; you hear a scream, and you know that a poor creature who objects to its fate has slipped from his hand and is making its way among the crowd. You pass on and if you dare, you go up Black Hall Court or some of the other courts hard by, and you feel your heart sink within you to think of the squalor and tragedy of the home life that can be possible in such surroundings.

The journalist who ventured into St Ann's Court went on to investigate a backyard in Berwick Street where he found a cesspool, a rubbish dump and a dirty sink. Climbing the ladder at the back of the house that served as the means of access to the first floor, he discovered two elderly women who told him that two people had died there and that the smell was particularly bad in their room because it was over a water-closet with no ceiling. The dogged reporter then clambered down into the base-ment where he found another old woman who earned her living by mangling washing. 'Here you see sir I am obliged to live,' she told him. 'I pay 3s a week rent. I have a mangle and cannot very well leave my bread [that is, her means of earning a living], but you see the floor is rotten and the smell at times is dreadful. When I sit by the fireplace, it is almost as bad as being in a water-closet.'

One step up the economic ladder from the basement dwellers came the skilled craftsmen, mostly tailors, milliners and wig-makers who supplied the gentlemen's outfitters and the luxury gown shops of Bond Street and Regent Street, and who made up most of the residents. Their living conditions were not much better than the washerwoman's, and in his 1842 inquiry into the lives of the working classes, Edwin Chadwick revealed that their places of work were nearly as bad. Fifty-two-year-old Thomas Brownlow had worked at some of the largest tailoring shops in London, including eight years at Messrs Allens of Old Bond Street. There, eighty tailors were crammed into a room measuring about seven-teen yards by eight yards, said Brownlow; their only source of daylight for the close work that usually ruined their eyesight, a pane of glass in the roof. 'The men were close together, nearly knee to knee,' Brownlow recalled. 'In summer time the heat of the men and the heat of the irons made the room twenty or thirty degrees higher than the heat outside . . .' The men started work at 6 a.m. and finished at 7 p.m., keeping going through the day with the help of snuff, beer and gin.

Apart from the tailors, the Soho residents consisted of local traders – publicans, cheesemongers, egg merchants, bakers and greengrocers – together with a motley collection of barbers, under-takers, policemen, laundresses, bricklayers, cabinet-makers and french polishers. Even among the steady wage-earners, though, whole families still often lived in a single room, or even part of a room, in an elegant but decaying house. Henry Whitehead asked one of his parishioners how on earth she managed to live at such close quarters with her fellow tenants. 'Well, sir,' came the answer. 'We was comfortable enough till the gentleman came in the middle.' The curate then realised the significance of the chalk circle in the centre of the room: it marked the floor space that 'the gentleman in the middle' called home.

It was little better out in the lanes. 'Throughout all the neigh-bourhood, the inhabitants complain greatly of smells in the streets,' Hall's men reported. 'In one case the offensive smell was arising from the tripe-boiling establishment and slaughter house in Marshall Street; also from the smell of the fermenting grains, usually kept in large quantities in the cow-yard adjoining the latter place . . . and from several of the fishmongers' shops and yards.' They were also concerned about the many small slaughterhouses where sheep and cows were killed in stuffy kitchen basements, and about the 'accumulations of imperfectly cleaned bones' left lying around by the district's many dealers in rags, grease and other recycled refuse.

But the worse smells of all came from the drains, privies and cesspits, which were constantly overflowing into the streets and yards or sometimes, in the case of the cesspits, up through the cellars. Few of the cesspits had ever been drained, and no one was even entirely sure where they all were any more. A shoemaker at number 5 South Row said that the stench from a nearby drain was so great 'as to compel him frequently to shut his window, and when he was desirous of opening it for a short time, he had recourse to the expedient of covering the grating with a piece of oil cloth with stones laid on it,' according to Hall's inspectors. Gutter pipes were also 'a fruitful source of foul smells, more particularly in those cases where the occupants of the attics are able to empty their slops into the roof gutters'. The occupant of the top floor of number 38 Silver Street went further. He kept twenty-seven dogs in one room, 'their excrements being discharged into the gutter on the roof where they accumulated and were described as emitting a horrible stench'.

It says much about the social conditions of the urban poor that this district was thought to be perfectly reasonable as far as working-class London was concerned and a definite cut above those areas considered really deprived, such as the nearby St Giles or the infamous district known as Jacob's Island in Bermondsey, South London, where Bill Sykes met his end in *Oliver Twist*.

Despite the living conditions in Broad Street then, people wondered why this area had been singled out for such a vicious attack. Perhaps something more than ordinarily unpleasant might be going on? Scare stories started to spread about a plague pit where the victims of another devastating disease had been laid to rest some 200 years before. The site had long since been covered with houses, and earlier that year when a new sewer was laid through part of Soho, people in Cambridge Street and Silver Street had watched fascinated as the workmen dug up piles of black bones. Some of the local boys had earned 2s a day selling the remains to the rag and bone dealers, and one family in Silver Street claimed that their health had never been the same since. Were these the bones of the plague victims? And by disturbing them had the authorities unwittingly released poison into the air?

Inspectors Fraser, Hughes and Ludlow, however, suspected that some of those putting forward the plague-pit theory might have an ulterior motive. One of the sewer's most vociferous critics, for example, was James Holmes, owner of the Marshall Street slaughterhouse and tripe-boiling works that were such a constant source of complaint. So-called 'nuisance' traders like Holmes were keen to ensure that when it came to apportioning the blame for this episode, no one would be looking in their direction. When the authorities checked up on the exact whereabouts of the burial ground, they found that the site was some distance from where local rumour had placed it and it didn't match the epicentre of the outbreak. And the engineer Joseph Bazalgette, who was to be responsible for the magnificent drainage system that still serves London today, wrote that the streets dug up by his workmen had in fact suffered the fewest casualties from cholera.

Eighteen months earlier at the end of 1852, as Snow's career as an anaesthetist at last took off, he had moved from his apartment in Frith Street, off Soho Square, to a better address in Sackville Street, Piccadilly. Thanks to a comfortable income, the Yorkshire labourer's son now had a spacious eighteenth-century house to himself, along with a resident housekeeper. Professionally he had achieved some success since his student days at Bateman's Buildings with Joshua Parsons, but he was still living just minutes' walk from Broad Street.

When Snow left his 'Grand Experiment' unfinished in south London that first week in September, cholera in Soho was out of control. One of his first actions was to go again to William Farr's Registrar General's Office for more statistics – this time for the cholera deaths in the sub-districts of Golden Square, Berwick Street and St Ann's, Soho. He studied the figures carefully. For the week ending the previous Saturday, 2 September, eighty-nine deaths had been reported, eighty-three of them on the Thursday, Friday and Saturday. This did not include people who had died in hospital or those whose deaths hadn't yet been registered: the final total for the three days would be 197.

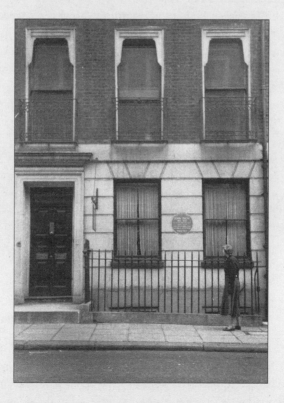

John Snow's house at 18 Sackville Street, London,
now demolished

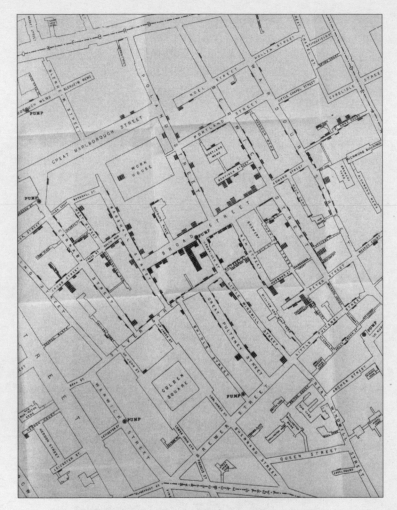

John Snow's 'disease map' of the Broad Street epidemic.
Each death is shown as a black line

As with south London, Snow then looked at the addresses where the fatal cases had occurred but this time he went further, and in so doing he made use of what is now a vital tool in the science of epidemiology, disease-mapping. He marked the deaths, house by house, on a street plan, a line for each fatality. And as he did so, a distinct pattern began to emerge. The map certainly showed just how local the outbreak was – confined almost entirely to a tiny clutch of streets, with the lines of the deaths appearing as thick black blocks against so many of the houses – but to Snow's keen eye, something else stood out, both figuratively on the map and physically on Broad Street, right at the heart of the outbreak and, to his way of thinking, as obvious a culprit as could be. He made his way over to Broad Street, passing as he went the houses where so many people had died or were dying even then. There on the corner with Cambridge Street outside number 40 where the Lewis family lived and a few doors down from the Eley percussion cap factory where eighteen people lost their lives, stood the Broad Street pump.

The night of Sunday, 3 September, found John Snow at home in Sackville Street studying samples of the pump water under his microscope. He expected to find large quantities of rotting organic matter, but to his surprise the water looked pure and clear. Had he made a mistake, after all, in suspecting that the fault lay with the pump? In order to find the answer, he took to the streets once again and began making some inquiries about the people who had died. His instincts were to trust the evidence from epidemiology rather than microbiology – in other words what was actually happening on the ground rather than what the microscope seemed to show.

According to his map, only ten deaths had taken place in houses that were clearly nearer to another pump: either the one in Rupert Street to the south or that in Berners Street, north of Oxford Street, where Dr Rogers lived. Rupert Street was misleading in that the road was a cul-de-sac and the pump stood hard by the dead end. 'With regard to the pump in Rupert Street, it will be noticed that some streets which are near to it on the map, are in fact a good way removed, on account of the circuitous road to it,' Snow pointed out. Five of the ten victims' families told Snow that their relative had preferred the water from Broad Street and always used that pump. Three of the other victims were children who went to school near Broad Street and were known to drink from the pump as they passed.

In the two remaining cases he found no link with Broad Street, but statistically this was in line with the existing mortality rate in the area since the national epidemic hit London earlier that summer. Twenty-six cases had been registered in the Berwick Street and Golden Square areas up to 30 August, and Snow regarded the events of the night of the 31 August and the days that followed not as a new outbreak, but rather as a particularly violent explosion of an already existing one.

Setting aside those victims who drank the Broad Street water even though the pump was not the nearest to their homes, the map clearly showed that the deaths had either plummeted or stopped altogether at every point where it was easier to go to another pump than the one in Broad Street. 'The wide open street in which the pump is situated suffered most,' Snow revealed, 'and next the streets branching from it, and especially those parts of them which are nearest to Broad Street. If there have been fewer deaths in the southern half of Poland Street than in some other streets leading from Broad Street, it is no doubt because this street is less densely inhabited.'

The result of Snow's foot-in-the-door investigation was the discovery that in sixty-one cases out of the eighty-three, the victim either always or sometimes drank from the pump. In six cases he couldn't get any information because anyone who knew anything about the victim was either dead themselves or had fled. As for the remaining victims who were thought not to have touched the pump water, they could easily have taken it without themselves or their friends knowing, Snow learnt. All of the pubs used it to mix with spirits, and it was on the table in every local dining-room and coffee shop. 'The keeper of a coffee shop in the neighbourhood, which was frequented by mechanics and where the pump water was supplied at dinner time, informed me that she was already aware of nine of her customers who were dead,' Snow reported. 'The pump water was also sold in various little shops with a tea-spoonful of effervescing powder in it under the name of sherbet; and it may have been distributed in various other ways with which I am unacquainted.'

It also transpired that the army officer from St John's Wood had washed down his Wardour Street dinner with water from the same source just hours before he died, and that the mother from Bentinck Street had gone to Broad Street for water the day before the family fled to Gravesend. And in the case of Mr Wickwar from Brighton, who had arrived too late to attend the deathbed of his brother John, the finger of suspicion pointed firmly at that small glass of brandy and water that he threw hurriedly down his throat on his way out of the house, the water in question having come from the Broad Street pump.

No matter how innocent that water might appear under the microscope, Snow could find no other possible link between the people who had died. And over the next few days, the specimens began to look more suspicious: he could make out some small, white, scaly particles, and the stuff smelt foul when it was left standing. Mr Eley, the proprietor of the percussion cap factory and son of Susannah who died in Hampstead, said that the con-tents of the jug he kept in his bedroom tasted like dead mice, and one or two people noticed a deterioration. The ornithologist John Gould, famous for his intricate illustrations of Australian birds, was one of the few professional people still living in the area. Gould was out of town when the outbreak began but as soon as he arrived home on the morning of Saturday, 2 September, he sent for some water. He didn't drink it, however, because although it looked harmless enough, it smelt horrible. Gould's assistant followed his master's example, but one of the servants had drunk from the pump on that fateful Thursday and had been among the first to be seized.

Nevertheless, the vast majority of local people had noticed nothing wrong at the time when the water was presumably at its most deadly, and this, coupled with his microscope's failure to reveal a problem, led Snow to a further conclusion. The amount of 'morbid matter' needed to produce the disease must be inconceivably small, he said, and consequently the shallow pump wells in daily use in towns and cities throughout the country must be regarded with great suspicion, however good their reputation for clean, pure water might be. No one paid the slightest attention to this.

Then, crucially, he went much further by managing to solve some mysteries that seemed, on the face of it, to undermine his theory. The great workhouse in Poland Street, where Snow sometimes gave anaesthesia in the infirmary, stood right in the middle of the danger zone surrounded by dozens of houses where people had died, yet lost only five of its 535 inmates. Snow discovered that the institution never took water from Broad Street; it had its own pump-well on the premises and also a supply from the Grand Junction Water company, an arrangement which Snow calculated had saved over a hundred lives.

Another strange story concerned the Lion Brewery; this was situated just a few yards from the pump and yet not one of its workers died. Snow described how he found the answer to this particular puzzle:

> I called on Mr. Huggins, the proprietor, who informed me that there were above 70 workmen employed in the brewery, and that none of them had suffered from cholera – at least in a severe form – only two having been indisposed, and that not seriously. The men are allowed a certain quantity of malt liquor, and Mr. Huggins believes they do not drink water at all, and he is quite certain that the workmen never obtained water from the pump in the street.

Snow, of course, was not the only man to be out on the streets of Soho looking for answers. Also on the trail were Hall's officials, armed with their bundles of forms on which to record the information that their masters back in Whitehall were demanding. Driven by a miasmatist agenda, the inspectors were looking at a much wider range of factors than Snow – including smells, drains and even the victims' alcohol consumption. Ironically, it was a member of this government team who led John Snow to the information that was to prove conclusive.

In the register of births and deaths for the week ending 9 September, David Fraser spotted a death in the district of Hampstead, to the north-west of London and several miles from Soho: 'At West End, on 2nd September, the widow of a percussion-cap maker, aged 59 years, diarrhoea two hours, cholera epidemic 16 hours.' This was Susannah Eley, widow of William, who had moved from Soho to Hampstead and whose family's detonator factory at 37 Broad Street was now run by her sons. Susannah had died on the second day of the Soho epidemic, although she hadn't been near the district in months, and the niece visiting her had died the day after. Investigating a death in Hampstead was not part of Dr Fraser's brief, but he passed this curious detail on to Snow, who went to talk to one of the young Mr Eleys. He was told that the firm always kept two large tubs of pump water in the yard for thirsty employees, which explained why eighteen workers had died.

But there was something else much more interesting: 'I was informed by this lady's son that she had not been in the neighbourhood of Broad Street for many months but a cart went from Broad Street to West End every day, and it was the custom to take out a large bottle of the water from the pump in Broad Street, as she preferred it. The water was taken on Thursday, 31 August, and she drank of it in the evening, and also on Friday. She was seized with cholera on the evening of the latter day and died on Saturday. A niece, who was on a visit to this lady, also drank of the water. She returned to her residence in a high and healthy part of Islington, was attacked with cholera and died also. There was no cholera at the time either at West End or in the neighbourhood where the niece died.' When Snow had published his first cholera paper in 1849, the *London Medical Gazette* had said that the key test of his theory would be to show that water 'conveyed to a distant and unaffected locality would produce the disease in all who drank it'. Here was the proof.

Snow's final conclusion was that there had been no particular increase of cholera in the area except among those who were in the habit of drinking water from the Broad Street well. He was now convinced beyond any doubt that the water was the one and only cause of the whole tragedy. 'Whilst the presumed contamination of the water of the Broad Street pump with the evacuations of cholera patients affords an exact explanation of the fearful outbreak of cholera in St James's parish, there is no other circumstance which offers any explanation at all, whatever hypothesis of the nature and cause of the malady be adopted,' he wrote.

So on the evening of Thursday, 7 September, he made his way to the Vestry Hall in Piccadilly, less than a minute's walk from his home in Sackville Street, and asked for permission to address the meeting of the Board of Guardians of St James's Parish, Westminster, that was currently under way. Carefully he explained his investigations to the parishmen and told them what he wanted them to do – they must take the handle off the Broad Street pump. The Guardians listened open-mouthed. Who was this strange fellow who had turned up unannounced with such a bizarre story to tell?

They really didn't find him at all convincing.

CHAPTER 14

Euglenae and Red Cotton

Many of the public believe that everything we eat and drink teams with life and that even our bodies abound with minute living and parasitic productions. This is a vulgar error and the notion is as disgusting as it is erroneous

Arthur Hill Hassall, Report of the Committee for Scientific Inquiry, 1855

Sir Benjamin Hall's Medical Council, like his inspectors on Broad Street, lost no time in starting work. With a cholera outbreak liable to stop as abruptly as it had started, it was vital to have the research underway while the evidence was still to hand. Letters went out to medical men throughout the capital and beyond calling for reports on the treatments they had used and to what effect, while the experts in chemistry, microscopy and meteorology set about their varied investigations.

The microscopist, Arthur Hill Hassall, took water samples from all over London, both from the supplies of the different companies and the contents of many of the pump wells. Subjecting them all to close examination, his findings were replicated in a series of delicate and beautiful hand-coloured drawings, depicting myriad creatures, both grotesque and marvellous. The artist was the same Mr Miller who accompanied Hassall on his nightly shopping trips on behalf of the Analytical Sanitary Commission and illustrated the results for the *Lancet*.

Not surprisingly, given John Snow's research, one of Hassall's conclusions was that the outpourings of the Southwark and Vauxhall company – still taking its supplies from the most polluted part of the Thames and responsible, according to Snow, for large numbers of cholera deaths in south London – were the filthiest in the capital. Southwark and Vauxhall water 'swarmed with living organic productions of various kinds,' said Hassall, adding, 'It is clear that this is a highly impure water and is wholly unfit for use as a beverage.' The microscopist said he could have filled an entire volume with the descriptions of the different species swimming around in one sample from a house near Albion Terrace.

The Chelsea Company's water contained the same organisms, Hassall found, which was hardly surprising seeing that Chelsea took its supply from almost the same part of the river as Southwark and Vauxhall. But because Chelsea at least bothered to filter its product before piping it into Londoners' homes, the numbers of animalcules were 'greatly diminished'.

By 9 September, ten days after the start of the Broad Street outbreak, Hassall and the chemist Robert Thomson were in Soho taking samples from those houses with their own water supply. Many people who had piped water still used the pumps, however, because commercial supplies were spasmodic to say the least. At 3 South Row, where two families shared one basement room and where three people had died, Hassall reported that the piped water contained the following extras:

Two or three euglenae, several of brown rolling lenticular animalculae, which I cannot identify with any described in works, and two or three other minute infusoria. The residue which collected at the bottom of the glass was not inconsiderable and there were present anguillula fluviatilis, four or five rotifers, one paramecium, a great many of the productions known as pandorina morum in all stages of growth, a few of the peculiar brown rolling bodies referred to above, scenedesmus quadricauda, a great many frustules of synedra and naviculae and a few of the diatoma, asterionella formosa.

Hassall and Thomson also tested patients' blood, urine, skin and clothes and, as the Bristol doctors had done before them, the so-called 'rice-water evacuations'. For the latter samples, Hassall had his microscope ready and waiting in the Abernethy Ward of St Bartholomew's Hospital, and when the two scientists peered through their instruments they were intrigued to find 'myriads' of what Hassall called *vibriones* – by which he meant elongated, motile micro-organisms – 'in every drop of every sample of rice water discharges hitherto subjected to examination'. He went on: 'It appears that vibriones are constantly present in cholera discharges and that they are developed in it during life and while still retained in the small intestine. Without however at all supporting that there is any essential or primary connection between these vibriones and cholera, their occurrence in such vast numbers . . . is not without interest and possibly of importance.' Mystery still surrounds the Bristol doctors' findings, but Hassall's descriptions leave little doubt about what he had stumbled upon. His failure to investigate further – despite describing the presence of huge numbers of 'vibriones' as 'possibly of importance' – and to establish that there was indeed a primary connection between the *vibriones* and cholera, lost him an exalted place in medical history. His big mistake was to assume that the *vibriones* in question were the result of the disease, rather than its cause.

As a chemist, Robert Thomson had been considering how best to analyse the air exhaled by cholera patients and to this end he developed an ingenious 16 cubic-foot, zinc-lined wooden tank that used suction in order to pull air through a trap of distilled water. Positioning this contraption in a cholera ward at St Thomas's Hospital, he then took samples when the ward was full of patients, when it was half full and when it was empty. He also took samples of air from the street and the sewer. When he examined them under the microscope, he found that the air from the cholera ward contained: 'blue and red cotton, hair, wool, sporules, fungi in very early and advanced stages of development, vibriones and particles of silica and dirt'.

The meteorologist James Glaisher also spared no efforts in his attempts to help Hall's cause. His final report contained no fewer than sixty-two tables and charts, showing atmospheric pressure, air and river temperatures, humidity, wind directions, wind forces, air velocity, atmospheric electricity, rain clouds, ozone and what he called 'atmospheric phenomena in the cholera districts'. Much of the data was based on comprehensive readings taken at meteorological stations all over central London and its outlying districts, from the Royal Observatory, Greenwich – presided over by no less a personage than the Astronomer Royal – to one at Enfield vicarage faithfully manned by the Reverend Heath.

In the meantime, reports flooded in from medical men throughout the country describing a wide range of treatment regimens, most involving brandy, opium and calomel in various combinations and dosages, while the results of a series of post-mortems on cholera victims were carefully written up for inclusion.

The result was a mass of scientific data on everything from the weather to the state of the victims' kidneys, but quite what the Medical Council was supposed to make of it all was far from clear. Sir Benjamin Hall had been understandably determined to leave no possible factor unexamined, but the huge scope of this inquiry left those attempting to interpret the findings with a Herculean task. Nor was their work helped by the fact that they were convinced miasmatists to a man – which left them completely unable to recognise a few startlingly clear clues under their noses.

CHAPTER 15

The Verdicts

"Dr Snow's views on cholera," said a medical friend to me in 1855, "are generally regarded in the profession as very unsound." "If that be the case," I replied, "then heresy may be as good a thing in your profession as some of you are apt to suppose it is in mine."

Reverend Henry Whitehead

It was a measure of their desperation that the parishmen agreed to John Snow's request, even though no one in the hall in Piccadilly that September night had ever heard of him or his theory, and not one of them seriously believed that he might be right. Still, with the bodies of their fellow citizens being trundled off by the cart-load, the guardians had little to lose, and consequently the very next day the handle came off the Broad Street pump. The myth has it that cholera was stopped dead in its tracks and that overnight Snow's theory was proved beyond dispute. Sadly though for those still to die in future epidemics, the reality was rather different.

Snow's intervention had come just a few days too late, and cholera was yet again one jump ahead of the game. By the time Snow had finished his enquiries and put his case to the guardians, the epidemic had peaked of its own accord. This was the shortest and sharpest of attacks. On 2 September, there had been 116 newly diagnosed cases that would prove fatal and 127 deaths. By 4 September, the new fatal cases were down to forty-six and the deaths down to seventy-one, and by 7 September, the day of the guardians' meeting, the figures were twenty-eight and thirty-two respectively. The source of the contamination, whatever it was, had dried up, and the well, which was only about 30 feet deep, had been quickly flushed clean, ironically by the local residents drinking its deadly contents. And, of course, there were far fewer people around since so many had died or fled the district. The situation was still, maddeningly, at stalemate.

One of the members of the St James's vestry, the body that held the parish purse-strings, was a doctor called Edwin Lankester who lived in Berwick Street near St Luke's Church. Lankester was a warm, loud and charismatic character who had fought his way up from a humble background largely through charm and determination, and despite being snubbed by the medical elite at the Royal College of Physicians. Behind his sociable, ebullient manner and a shambling incompetence over his finances that was to dog him all his days, lay a serious scientific mind and a fierce sense of social justice. He and Snow were very different personalities but they were the same age, came from similar lowly backgrounds, and shared the same devotion to the harnessing of science to improve the lives of their fellow men. By 1854 at the age of forty, Lankester was also a knowledgeable naturalist and an experienced microscopist.

For all that, Lankester didn't believe Snow any more than anyone else did. He thought that drinking bad water might have a part to play in making people more vulnerable to cholera, but only along with other risk factors such as drunkenness and individual susceptibility. The main culprit, he was sure, was the gases given off by rotting animal and vegetable matter, in other words, miasma. As a doctor and a vestryman, Lankester felt he had a dual responsibility to act, particularly as his parish had been so maddeningly slow to respond when the outbreak first struck and, like Sir Benjamin before him, he thought hard about the problem before coming up with a plan that he thought might help to navigate a way through what the *Lancet* had recently described as the 'whirlpool of conjecture' over the causes of cholera.

At a vestry meeting on 2 November, a little over a month after the epidemic subsided, Lankester proposed that the parish hold its own inquiry into the tragedy, and accordingly a committee of vestrymen under Lankester's chairmanship was appointed for the task. When the board of guardians heard what was going on they were furious and wrote to express their 'dissatisfaction and alarm'. Presumably they were expected to pay for this piece of self-indulgence? Where was the money to come from? The poor rate certainly couldn't be expected to bear the cost and, more to the point, what on earth did the vestry think it was doing by dragging all this up again now, just as the government officials had finally finished their prying and local businesses were starting to recover from the terrible publicity? It took all of Lankester's powers of persuasion to stop his committee being wound up before it started work. They were then snubbed by Sir Benjamin Hall, who refused to let them see the material the government team was collecting on the grounds that the parishmen's investigation would be all the better if they did the work for themselves.

Soon after setting up, Lankester invited some outsiders to join the ranks, notably John Snow, whom Lankester knew through the Westminster Medical Society, and the twenty-nine-year-old curate from St Luke's Church in Berwick Street, Henry Whitehead, who had won his right to a committee seat by publishing a pamphlet, 'The Cholera in Berwick Street', just weeks after the epidemic. The priest had concentrated on describing what had happened during those few days the previous summer rather than specu- lating on the causes, but he believed that the scientists had a sacred duty to investigate. 'There was evidently something new and distinct that suddenly came into operation during the very last hours of that month [of August, 1854],' he wrote. 'What that was, it is to be hoped that those who have knowledge of such matters will endeavour to ascertain. The writer believes that we shall not be discharging our duty, either before our fellow men or the All-wise Ruler of the Universe, unless we make the most strenuous exertions for this purpose.'

Unlike both Snow and Lankester, Whitehead had been raised in comfortable circumstances in Ramsgate, Kent, where his father was a master at a small public school. Despite an elite education at Lincoln College, Oxford, Whitehead, in contrast to the painfully shy John Snow, had the common touch in huge measure. Sociable and hospitable, he loved nothing more than to have a group of friends round to dinner at his lodgings in Soho Square or to spend the evening in a pub. Ye Old Cheshire Cheese off Fleet Street was one of his favourites. 'He found an occasional dinner at a London tavern good for both body and soul,' remarked one of his friends, adding: 'There was a strong Johnsonian element in his composition, and the book of human nature was what he preferred to any other.'

The curate's friendliness and kindness made him a welcome visitor in homes throughout his parish, and his fellow priest Harry Jones described how during the 'deadly slaughter', when the yellow warning flags flew at one end of Berwick Street, and the hearses rumbled out of the other, Whitehead had 'fought like a hero night and day, with hand and lips and brain, helping to strengthen the living, heal the sick and comfort the dying'. 'I can't say I saw much of Whitehead then for we both had our hands full,' remembered Jones, 'but one thought of the man in the thickest of the fight.'

As with many priests working in the slums of the day, Whitehead's role combined spiritual guidance with the pragmatic work of a community social worker long before the latter profession existed. And while he loved the people he had come to serve, he had no illusions about the lowly part that religion played for many of them in their daily struggle for existence. He delighted in repeating a conversation overheard between two poverty-stricken women: 'And how do you get on this winter?' asked one. 'Very poorly indeed,' replied the other. 'There'll soon be nothing for it but to take to morning prayers.'

In January 1855 John Snow published his definitive work on cholera. Officially this is the second edition of his 1849 pamphlet, but the now classic, bound volume of 'On the Mode of Communication of Cholera' of 1855 is, at over 40,000 words, six times the length of the first version and contains a mass of new or expanded evidence and careful argument. Snow's central points – that cholera is contagious, that it is primarily a disease of the intestines and that it is spread by the oral-fecal route, largely through polluted water – remain unchanged, but he now backs this with an enormous body of material from Britain and India. With no direct microbiological evidence available to him, and in the days before Pasteur demonstrated the link between germs and disease, the work is based almost entirely on epidemiological deduction and all the more impressive for that. Snow also answers all of the big questions that Sir Benjamin Hall had asked his experts to address.

He begins with what was then known about the history of the disease from its origins in India and goes on to state that cholera is clearly passed from person to person, backing this up with dozens of examples. He then considers how cholera affects the body – maintaining again that this is a disease whose 'poison' must be swallowed; and discusses the analyses of patients' blood and evacuations carried out by Edmund Parkes of University College Hospital, to whom he first mentioned his ideas in 1848. He argues, correctly, that Parkes's results show that the thick, tarry state of the victims' blood is a direct result of the diarrhoea and vomiting. Then comes a huge amount of evidence to show that cholera is transmitted through polluted water, not only through the accounts of events at Horsleydown and Albion Terrace but with other examples of outbreaks in Rotherhithe, Manchester, Ilford, Bath, Newcastle, Deptford, at Cunnatore in India and among the French and British fleets on the Black Sea.

The outbreak in Broad Street, which of course happened five years after the publication of the first edition of 'On the Mode of . . .', merits its own section, and Snow tells the story of Soho with some verve, grabbing the reader's attention with his first sentence: 'The most terrible outbreak of cholera which ever occurred in this kingdom, is probably that which took place in Broad Street, Golden Square, and the adjoining streets, a few weeks ago.' He then goes on to trace the course of the disease, recount anecdotes, describe case histories from the books of local doctors, set out statistics and reproduce his now famous map of the streets where the deaths occurred. Most importantly though, and with his usual step-by-step logic, he sets out his reasons for blaming the Broad Street pump, dealing along the way with those strange cases that seemed, on the face of it, to mitigate against him but in fact add greater weight to his case, such as the death of Susannah Eley, the Hampstead widow, and the apparent immunity of the workers at the Lion brewery.

Snow next turns his attention to the water supply generally, and the part that this had played in three national epidemics, again backed by substantial evidence. Here he presents his tour de force – what is now known as the 'Grand Experiment' – comparing cholera deaths in households supplied by the South and Vauxhall and Lambeth water companies during the epidemics of 1848–9 and 1854, and showing the clear fall in the risk to Lambeth's customers after the company had moved its intake upstream, out of reach of the sewage of London.

In his final section, Snow says that while many doctors now appeared to accept that water had some part to play in deaths from cholera, they remained unconvinced that the disease was passed on from person to person through the 'morbid matter' being swallowed, either in drinking water or in some other way. Rather, they saw polluted water as a predisposing cause of the disease; in other words, it predisposed, or prepared, a person's system to be acted upon by some unknown cause, probably something in the atmosphere. But, Snow insists, 'opinion cannot long halt here,' and adds: 'If the effect of contaminated water be admitted, it must lead to the conclusion that it acts by containing the true and specific cause of the malady.'

He then gives an expanded version of his 1849 advice about personal hygiene and clean drinking water that he rightly thought necessary for the prevention, not only of cholera but of all other diseases capable of being spread in the same way. Here he correctly includes dysentery and typhoid, but then, rarely for him, over-reaches himself in what appears almost an afterthought by wrongly listing malaria, yellow fever and plague.

Snow goes on to urge the government to have confidence in the British public and not to hide the 'true facts' about contagion from them. 'The communicability of cholera ought not to be disguised from the people under the idea that the knowledge of it would cause a panic or occasion the sick to be deserted,' he writes.

British people would not desert their friends or relatives in illness, [even] though they should incur danger by attending to them; but the truth is, that to look on cholera as a "catching" disease, which one may avoid by a few simple precautions, is a much less discouraging doctrine than that which supposes it to depend on some mysterious state of the atmosphere in which we are all of us immersed and obliged to breathe.

He ends by saying that any preventative measures must be based on correct information; in the past ignorance had often led to people making matters worse, and here Snow refers to Edwin Chadwick's frantic flushing of London's sewers into the Thames during the 1848–9 epidemic. He adds: 'I feel confident that by attending to the above-mentioned precautions . . . this disease may be rendered extremely rare, if indeed it may not be altogether banished from civilized countries.'

This second edition of 'On the Mode of . . .' received slightly more publicity than the first but not much, and it was hardly a best-seller. Snow's hopes can't have been high on this score, however, given his experience to date, and he clearly had his tongue firmly in his cheek when he wrote in the preface: 'I feel confident that my present labours will receive the same kind consideration from the medical profession which has been accorded to my former endeavors to ascertain the causes of cholera.' The *Lancet* finally reviewed it nearly a year after publication; and while conceding that experience over the years had by now shown that cholera could be communicated from person to person, the journal was sceptical about Snow's claim that this was a disease of the digestive system and noncommittal about his views on the role of drinking water.

'On the Mode of' cost John Snow over £200 to print, and he was later to complain that its total sales earnt him less than 200 shillings. He sent Henry Whitehead a complimentary copy, but the curate was unconvinced by what he read, particularly about Broad Street. If the blame was with the pump, then the contamination must be coming from the sewer that ran close to the well, or so Whitehead assumed. However, the sewer was new and unlikely to leak, and even if it had leaked, why did the epidemic stop so suddenly at a time when dozens of people living on the line of that sewer were suffering from cholera and, presumably, adding to the pollution of the water? Whitehead first wrote to Snow explaining his views and then he set off on a one-man mission, using his local knowledge and every opportunity that his work among the poor afforded him to question every family about their living conditions and how they had been affected by the cholera. He was determined to prove Snow wrong, and he told a friend that the task would be an easy one. It was not.

He travelled long distances to trace people who had left the district, and went back to see others four or five times as he thought of vital questions he had forgotten to ask the first time round. There was also great difficulty in getting people to remember the exact turn of events during those confused, frightening days. In one household, the only person who could recall what had happened was a very old man who was somewhat deaf. Whitehead found himself conducting a bellowed conversation about the circumstances surrounding a particular glass of gin and water drunk on a particular night in September six months earlier with an individual whose memory was as keen as his hearing was defective. The diligent curate then hit upon the idea of holding group interviews, and began assembling local mothers together for in-depth discussions of their families' drinking habits. 'This method possessed the obvious advantage of their assisting and correcting each other's evidence,' he explained.

For four months Henry Whitehead worked well into the night painstakingly compiling his dossier, and as he did so a surprising picture began to emerge. Far from refuting Snow's theory, to his astonishment the curate found himself confirming it, even when at first the facts appeared to go against Snow. On one occasion Whitehead went to see a couple with a baby and a little girl of ten. They had moved out of the district on 4 September and had only just returned.

> I asked whether any of them had been attacked with cholera or diarrhoea? No. Were they in the habit of using the pump water? Yes. Who fetched it? The little girl. Was she not afraid, I then asked the child, of going through the streets and seeing the shutters all up and so many hearses about? Didn't go through the streets. Why not? Was ill in bed with a cold. I asked the mother whether that was the case. She then called to mind that it was so. Who fetched the water then when the child was unable to go for it? Why then they got it from the cistern.

In fact, so many families were in the habit of sending the children to fetch water from the pump that Whitehead was finally able to make sense of a phenomenon that had been puzzling him for some time. Preaching a sermon at the height of the epidemic, he noticed that his much-depleted congregation consisted almost entirely of old women. He congratulated them on their strength in withstanding the disease but privately he found it very odd that they, of all people, should have escaped unscathed. Now the reason was clear: they lived alone and had no one to send to the pump. Slowly and reluctantly then, the curate admitted, he was drawn to the conclusion that the 'commencement and continuance of the outburst' was linked to the water from the Broad Street pump.

But then he went further and made a discovery that had eluded even John Snow. If the problem was indeed with the pump, then how had the water become infected? This was a question that remained unanswered at Tooting. A few cholera deaths had been registered in Soho earlier that summer before the main outbreak, but none of the known cases seemed to fit the facts. Whitehead wondered about a boy who arrived in Broad Street from Bayswater where the disease was prevalent and fell ill soon after, on 28 August. The timing was about right, the curate thought, but the house where the lad had been staying was more than thirty yards from the pump.

Just days before Whitehead was due to hand over his report to Lankester's committee, he happened to be looking through the registrars' returns of deaths for a reason quite unconnected with the epidemic when he noticed the following entry: 'At 40 Broad Street, 2nd September, a daughter, aged five months, exhaustion after an attack of diarrhoea four days previous to death.' This was Sarah Lewis's baby – the child Dr Rogers had treated and whose death he had certified – and whose father, PC Thomas Lewis, had died of cholera two weeks later. Whitehead knew the Lewis family well, but the significance of what had happened at number 40 didn't dawn on him until he read that entry. Now it was staring him in the face. The pump was right outside the house, and the child's fatal illness had started forty-eight hours before that terrible night of 31 August. His own research had shown him that, given a causal link with drinking contaminated water, this was the typical incubation period for cholera.

He hurried round to Broad Street to find Sarah Lewis, and she told him how she had soaked her sick baby's nappies in pails of water before tipping the contents into the cesspit at the front of the house: a cesspit that was less than three feet away from the pump well. When Whitehead reported this to the vestry, along with his growing conviction that John Snow was right, they ordered that the cesspit be examined. The local surveyor, Jehosephat York, duly instructed his men to dig down into the filthy sludge, just as Mr Grant's men had done at Albion Terrace in 1849. Neither Snow nor, by now, Henry Whitehead was surprised at what the labourers found. York reported:

The main drain of the house was opened in the front vault under the street and was found to be constructed on the old-fashioned plan of a flat bottom with brick sides and covered with old stone. As this drain had but a small fall or inclination outwards to the main sewer, the bottom was covered with an accumulation of soil deposit ... and upon cleaning away this soil, the mortar joints of the old stone bottom were found to be perished, as was all the jointing of the brick sides, which brought the brickwork into the condition of a sieve and through which the house drainage water must have percolated for a considerable period. [They then opened the back of the drain where they found the cesspit underneath a crude open privy.] Upon removing the soil, the brickwork of the cesspool was found to be in the same decayed condition as the drain ... the bricks were easily lifted from their beds without the least force, so that any fluid could readily pass through.

Finally York turned to the question of whether contamination from the drain or the cesspit could leak into the well supplying the Broad Street pump. 'From the bottom of the house drain down to the water line in the well, a vertical depth of 9ft 2in exists; and from the side of the drain horizontally to the outer side of the brick work of the well, there is only a space of 2ft 8ins, whilst the side wall of the vault adjoining the cesspool actually abuts upon it,' he explained. 'Thus, therefore, from the charged condition of the cesspool, the defective state of its brickwork and also that of the drain, no doubt remains upon my mind that constant percolation, and for a considerable period, had been conveying fluid matter from the drains into the well.' And in case doubt should remain upon anyone else's mind, York checked the well's lining and found it saturated with black liquid. The similarities with Albion Terrace were all too clear. Conditions in that middle-class Battersea street might have looked a world away from those in Broad Street, Soho, but hidden away under the ground the same unsavoury state of affairs prevailed.

Now, Whitehead reasoned, supposing that the Lewis child had
had cholera and not, as Dr Rogers had concluded, simple diarrhoea? If Rogers had been wrong, then here might lie the cause of
the whole massive outbreak – the index case, as epidemiologists
call it – and with it the deaths of over 600 people. And there was
more. If the cesspit at number 40 Broad Street were to blame, then
while removing the pump handle on 8 September had come too
late to help the victims of this outbreak, it had almost certainly
prevented another, for Sarah had soaked her husband's soiled linen
in pails of water and then thrown the slops into the cesspit, just
as she had done two weeks earlier with her baby's nappies. And
Thomas had fallen sick on 8 September, the very day Snow had
caused the pump to be put out of action.

One month before Whitehead's discovery, in March 1855, by a
strange chance, John Snow was able to explain his ideas personally
to the key figure in the cholera debate – whose team of doctors, scientists and health inspectors had just finished work on a huge
inquiry – the president of the Board of Health, Sir Benjamin Hall.
The main topic under debate this time was not cholera, however,
and Snow was there not at the invitation of the medical profession
nor the politicians, but at the request of a group generally regarded
as a public menace.

Sir Benjamin was chairing a parliamentary inquiry into the so-
called 'nuisance trades' with a view to legislating against the
'noxious gases' produced by businesses such as abattoirs and tan-
neries. By now Snow's ideas were slightly better known among those
who had a special interest in epidemic disease, although not more
widely accepted, and he appeared before the committee as an expert
witness for the 'offensive' traders; the bone-boilers, soap manufac-
turers, tallow melters, makers of chemical fertiliser and others who
were keen to show that there was nothing wrong with a few nasty
smells. It is unclear exactly how the tradesmen, or perhaps their
lawyer, heard about Snow, but it seems to have been late in the day
and by chance. He was approached by a bone merchant called
Henry Knight and at the last minute, for Snow mentions in passing

that he was only given a couple of days' notice. There is no record of whether he was paid, but he certainly spoke from conviction, although the MPs clearly had difficulty in believing their ears.

No one – including Sir Benjamin who was so interested in the mode of transmission of cholera – made any comment at all when Snow told them that he believed that cholera was spread mainly through drinking water, but when it came to his views on bad smells, they could not hide their astonishment. Snow told the committee:

I have arrived at the conclusion with regard to what are called offensive trades . . . that, in fact, they are not injurious to the public health. I consider that if they were injurious to the public health they would be extremely so to the workmen engaged in those trades, and, as far as I have been able to learn, that is not the case; and from the law of the diffusion of gases, it follows that if they are not injurious to those actually on the spot where the trades are carried on, it is impossible they should be to persons further removed from the spot.

'Are the committee to understand,' Sir Benjamin asked, 'taking the case of bone-boilers, that no matter how offensive to the sense of smell the effluvia that comes from bone-boiling establishments may be, yet you consider that it is not prejudicial in any way to the health of the inhabitants of the district?' 'That is my opinion,' was the simple answer.

And later: 'Do you not know that the effect of breathing such tainted air [that is, the smell of animal corpses or rotting vegetable matter] often is to produce violent sickness at the time?' 'Yes, when the gases are in a very large quantity, as in a cesspool.' 'Do you mean to tell the committee that when the effect is to produce violent sickness, there is no injury produced to the constitution or health of the individual?' 'No fever or special disease,' replied Snow.

The *Lancet*, true to form, had some colourful comments to

make. Those who opposed laws like that being proposed had vested interests 'in the production of pestilent vapours, miasms and loathsome abominations of every kind,' the journal announced, before going on to throw some of its finest invective at the manu-facturers' lobby: 'These unsavoury persons, trembling for the conservation of their right to fatten upon the injury of their neigh-bours, came in a crowd, reeking with putrid grease, redolent of stinking bones, fresh from seething heaps of stercoraceous deposits, to lay their "case" before the committee.'

In particular, the journal seized on the evidence of a soap-boiler, one Archibald Kintrea, who had told the MPs that he didn't think soap-boiling produced 'disagreeable effluvia'; on the contrary, he himself rather liked it and he thought that people generally enjoyed it, especially ladies. 'The odor of putrefying fat is not only salubri-ous but agreeable, if you can only make up your mind to discard vulgar prejudices,' mocked the Lancet. 'Some ladies live in an atmosphere of Eau de Cologne . . . others – Mr Kintrea's fair friends – dote upon the delicious fragrance of the copper when the soap-boiling is going on with intensity.'

And the soap-boiling Mr Kintrea was not the only person to be vilified by name. John Snow also came in for attack, in his case for bringing to the debate what the Lancet witheringly described as '"scientific" evidence!', the writer using punctuation to make clear that he thought Snow's views the very opposite of scientific. After accusing him of being blinded by his ideas, the journal goes on: 'Dr Snow claims to have discovered that the law of propagation of cholera is the drinking of sewage water. His theory, of course, dis-places all other theories. Other theories attribute great efficacy in the spread of cholera to bad drainage and atmospheric impuri-ties . . . The fact is that the well whence Dr Snow draws all sanitary truth is the main sewer. His specus, or den, is a drain. In riding his hobby very hard, he has fallen down through a gully-hole and has never since been able to get out again.' The journal ends with what was clearly intended as an amusing piece of sarcasm but was in fact a simple statement of truth: 'In that dismal Acherontic [infernal, gloomy] stream [i.e., the sewer] is contained the one and only true cholera germ and if you take care not to swallow that you are safe from harm. Smell it if you may, breathe it fearlessly but don't eat it.'

Snow did not reply.

But despite all the *Lancet*'s magnificent rantings and the MPs' incredulity at Snow's views, the resulting Nuisances Removal and Disease Prevention Act was in the end shaped by the weight of the vested interests that the *Lancet* so deplored. The nuisance traders were allowed to continue largely unchecked, while what Sir Benjamin Hall thought about John Snow is not recorded. Certainly Hall was later to accept the conclusions of his hand-picked team of medical scientists rather than those of a lone individual regarded by almost everyone who had heard of him as, at best, a maverick and, at worst, a crank with an obsession, but as a responsible politician, he could scarcely have done otherwise.

Meanwhile with the approach of another summer, Henry Whitehead noted that nerves in Soho were becoming frayed, and the curate felt the need to solve the mystery of the past year's tragedy more keenly than ever. 'A feeling of uneasy apprehension is beginning to prevail, even among those who have hitherto stood firm,' he wrote. 'Whenever the cholera shall reappear in the country, I have no doubt that this neighbourhood will be deserted by all who can conveniently depart, unless there shall previously have been given a satisfactory account of the causes of the late calamity and a reasonable prospect held out of the comparative immunity for the future.'

That July, Hall's illustrious Medical Council under the aegis of John Ayrton Paris, the president of the Royal College of Physicians, published the findings of its great study in the form of a volume consisting of four separate reports running to over 300 pages, together with a 350-page appendix complete with tables, figures and charts based on the researches of Thomson, Glaisher and

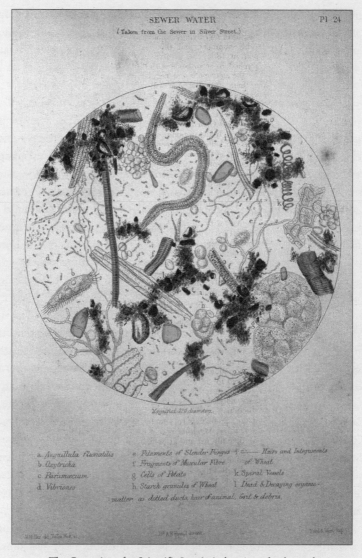

The Committee for Scientific Inquiry's drawing of a drop of
Soho sewer water, as seen under the microscope

Hassall. The Broad Street inspectors' twenty-eight-page report was included in full, together with the results of their house-to-house visits and a map showing, as John Snow's map showed, the houses where the deaths had occurred, as well as the sites of the supposed and the actual plague pit. The work was formally presented to both Houses of Parliament.

Ayrton Paris and his colleagues had made a valiant attempt to compare the effectiveness of different treatment regimens as described in the 2,750 case reports sent in by doctors around the country, and they drew up some guidelines for the future care of cholera patients. They advised against the use of emetics and purgatives, for example, and recommended that remedies such as ammonia, brandy and creosote should be used only in extreme cases, but they came out in favour of chalk and opium. Commending Ayrton Paris's view of laxatives, the *Lancet* remarked: 'This gives the final blow to that most irrational and fanciful of blunders – a blunder worthy only of a homeopathic brain – of seeking to arrest a disease of which the most fatal symptom is colliquative diarrhoea by the administration of agents having the effect of increasing diarrhoea.' Editor Wakley clearly had even more contempt for homeopaths than he did for the Royal College of Physicians. As it happened, Ayrton Paris and his colleagues were right about purgatives, but through luck rather than a correct interpretation of the data before them. In trying to assess and compare so many different treatments used in so many different combinations they had set themselves an impossible task, and there was never the slightest chance that they would be able to reach any meaningful conclusions.

But, of course, what really interested Sir Benjamin Hall was the attempt to track down the cause of the disease by studying the air, water and climate, and here his Committee for Scientific Inquiry – statistician William Farr, surgeon John Simon and the rest – had been deeply impressed by the meteorologist James Glaisher and his 'admirable system of observations'. Glaisher had gone a long way towards proving that the weather played an important part in epidemic mortality, they thought. In particular he had shown that in

1854, 1849 and, as far as anyone could tell, in 1832 too, the London climate had been ideal for encouraging the growth of poisonous matter in the air, and these conditions had increased and declined in line with the epidemics. 'Such facts accord well with the view that the poison of cholera enters the human body through the lungs,' Farr and his fellow experts announced.

In contrast to Glaisher's work, however, Robert Thomson's analyses of the air had proved a sad disappointment, despite his ingenious, purpose-built apparatus. His samples abounded with dust, common fungi and rotting organic matter, but there was nothing new or significant to be seen, and the experts' frustration was clear. 'We cannot pass this very interesting part of our subject without expressing our regret that researches of so much importance could not have been commenced at an earlier date and been made more comprehensive in their scope,' they wrote. 'A very complete and exact inquiry into the chemistry of organic decomposition during the epidemic prevalence of cholera – especially into the successful transformations of animal refuse at such times – might furnish all-important information as to the characteristic poison of the disease.' The evidence for the role of miasma was out there somewhere, they were clearly convinced; it was just a matter of finding it.

And there was a similarly inconclusive result from the investigations into drinking water. Hassall and Thomson had confirmed that the supplies in the shallow pump wells were bad, and those piped into London homes even worse, but neither had found anything specific that could be linked to cholera. Thomson had detected some chemical salts of a type usually associated with decomposing matter but there was no reason to think that consuming small doses of them would predispose anyone to disease, the experts said, and the same applied to the living organisms revealed by Hassall's microscope; the *euglenae*, the *anguillula fluviatilis*, the *pandorina morum* and the rest.

Parasites, the experts accepted, were often linked to disease, 'and for aught we know to the contrary, many of the creatures described by Dr Hassall may be capable of sustenance and multiplication within the bowels of those who swallowed them,' they wrote, 'but in every known case where it can be fairly presumed that parasites are the causes of disease, they exist as a palpable morbid product, occupying some considerable share of the affected body.' For example when a silkworm died from muscardine, its body was so riddled with the fungus that little remained but a heap of mould. Surely, then, in order for a parasite to induce cholera's violent symptoms, it would have to multiply in the gut in such swarms as to be obvious to the most casual observer? they reasoned.

'Again, in the intestinal discharges,' they went on, 'Dr Hassall has discovered no sporules or threads of any species of fungus, and no peculiar body of any kind other than *vibriones*.' The reason that they dismissed Hassall's *vibriones* so readily was partly because the microscopist himself had done so, but also because one of Thomson's colleagues had wrongly told them that these particular animalcules were commonly seen in patients with other diseases. Their presence in such huge numbers probably showed nothing more than 'a great proneness to decomposition' in cholera patients' guts, the experts thought. In other words, they agreed with Hassall that the *vibriones* were the result not the cause of the disease. Their own earlier comments that any cholera-causing animalcule would be seen swarming in the gut in huge numbers clearly rang no bells here.

And as far as Broad Street was concerned, here again the most painstaking investigations had drawn a blank. Inspectors Fraser, Hughes and Ludlow were completely unable to throw any light on why this area had been singled out for attack, despite their exhaustive street pounding and form filling. The whole affair was 'a difficulty which hitherto we have no scientific material to solve'.

Hall's experts then went on to single out an individual who was not used to the limelight. 'It has been suggested by Dr Snow that the real cause of whatever was peculiar in the case lay in the general use of one particular well situated at Broad Street and having its waters contaminated with the rice-water evacuations of cholera patients,' they began. Having raised the subject of Dr Snow, however, they were clearly keen to get him out of the way as quickly as possible. 'After careful inquiry we see no reason to adopt this belief. We do not find it established that the water was contaminated in the manner alleged, nor is there before us any sufficient evidence to show whether inhabitants in the district drinking from that well suffered in proportion more than other inhabitants of the district who drank from other sources.'

As for the death of Susannah Eley, whose only connection with Soho that previous summer had been a bottle of water from the Broad Street pump – an occurrence that even Edmund Parkes, no fan of John Snow's, described as 'the most extraordinary case which, if there is not some fallacy, is certainly unanswerable'– Hall's experts conceded that the water must have had some part to play but they had little difficulty in finding an explanation that satisfied their miasmatist agenda.

> The water was undeniably impure with organic contamination; and . . . if at the times of epidemic invasion, there be operating in the air some influence which converts putrefiable impurities into a specific poison, the water of the locality . . . would probably be liable to similar poisonous conversion. Thus, if the Broad Street pump did actually become a source of disease to persons dwelling at a distance . . . this . . . may have arisen, not in its containing choleraic excrements, but simply in the fact of its impure waters having participated in the atmospheric infection of the district.

The suddenness of the Soho attack and its short duration pointed to an 'atmospheric or other widely diffused agent still to be discovered,' they said, and they specifically ruled out person-to-person contagion 'either by infection or by contamination of water with the excretions of the sick'.

The final conclusion of Hall's eminent scientists then was that cholera was not a contagious disease but was caused by what they described as a 'wandering ferment' in the atmosphere that was activated into producing a cholera poison when it came into contact with foul air or water. No more telling example could be found of the grip that miasmatism had on the thinking of the country's medical elite than the findings of this government study, whose architect had had such faith in the ability of science to get to the truth.

On 9 August, Edwin Lankester presented the St James's parish with its own vestry committee's 175-page document, with separate reports by Whitehead, Snow and the surveyor Mr York. Lankester's committee had come up with a list of recommendations for their area. Shallow wells should no longer be used for drinking, and could perhaps be removed altogether and replaced with standpipes supplied from the mains. Cisterns, likewise, should go. Abattoirs, grease-boiling houses, bone stores and 'other offensive places of business' should be closed down and, whenever the opportunity arose, the many little cul-de-sacs and 'dead ends' throughout the district should be opened up to allow a better flow of air through the streets. And the parish should appoint a medical officer whose job it would be to warn the authorities about 'causes calculated to be detrimental to health which, under existing arrangements, lie dormant or accumulate to produce some unexpected and overwhelming calamity'. Given local attitudes to the spending of ratepayers' money, this was a somewhat unrealistic wish list, and they knew it.

On the cause of the cholera outbreak, however, while not issuing a resounding endorsement of John Snow, this little group, made up largely of local tradesmen, had decided that 'the sudden, severe and concentrated outbreak . . . was in some manner attributable to the use of the impure water of the well in Broad Street'. Six weeks later the Commissioners of Paving for the parish of St James bowed to pressure from local residents and reopened the pump.

By now Britain's third national cholera epidemic had petered out, and this time over 20,000 people had died. The small parish inquiry and the great government investigation had contributed two more tomes to the pile of volumes already written on the subject since 1817, yet neither had changed anything, or so it seemed. The following year, 1856, however, yet another official document on the subject saw the light of day. This one, a modest-looking pamphlet by John Simon, who had been on Hall's Committee for Scientific Inquiry and was now medical officer to the Board of Health, was entitled 'The Cholera Epidemics of London as Affected by the Consumption of Impure Water'. It turned out to be a virtual replica of John Snow's 'Grand Experiment', comparing death rates between the Lambeth and Southwark and Vauxhall water companies, but without a single reference to Snow or suggestion that the idea for the work had not been entirely Whitehall's. Simon, who stopped short of endorsing Snow's theory of the oral-fecal route for the spread of cholera, explained that this important piece of research was originally intended for inclusion in the original study but it had proved impossible to collate the results in time. John Snow made no complaint, but this time someone else had had enough.

Soon after Simon's publication appeared, Benjamin Ward Richardson stood up at a meeting of the British Medical Association, which Snow did not attend, to propose a motion of thanks to one Dr T. Bell Salter who had just given a talk on the laws of epidemics. But as well as expressing the audience's appreciation, Richardson said he felt compelled to point out what he was sure must have been an inadvertent slip on Dr Salter's part when he had referred to the Board of Health's work on the drinking water of south London. It was well known to anyone with an interest in this subject that the discovery of the connection between the water supply and cholera belonged solely to Dr John Snow. Indeed until recently the Board had completely ignored this vital question, and it was only when Dr Snow had 'with unwearied industry, with that genius for observation which so characterises his labours and at great pecuniary cost, placed the question beyond dispute . . . that the Board took up the matter'.

Richardson sat down to shouts of 'Hear hear' from the floor, and then another doctor rose from his seat to second everything that Richardson had said. He was Edwin Lankester, and he was followed by a third medical man, none other than William Budd, who along with Brittan and Swayne had been so badly discredited over the Bristol fungus affair in 1849. Budd could not let the occasion pass without expressing his entire agreement with Lankester and Ward, he told his colleagues. He had himself laboured over the question of the spread of cholera through contaminated drinking water, he said, but he was proud to have this opportunity to say that the entire priority of this investigation rested with Dr Snow.

Acclaim from a small group of doctors with a special interest in the spread of cholera was hardly the national recognition that John Snow's work deserved, but after all the years in the wilderness, it was something.

Two years later, on the evening of Wednesday, 9 June 1858, John Snow and Benjamin Ward Richardson attended a meeting of a society for the study of chest diseases at the London home of a colleague. Richardson was pleased to see how fit and cheerful his friend appeared, for he had been concerned about his health for some time. Snow had never been strong despite his love of fresh air and exercise, and had for some time had a foreboding that his life would not be a long one. As a young man he suffered from the bouts of exhaustion and the violent physical reaction to the slightest injury that had so worried Joshua Parsons. In his thirties he contracted tuberculosis and suffered from kidney problems, and in latter years had had episodes of vomiting blood, while a recent attack of giddiness and sickness had left him complaining of numbness in his hands and feet. That summer night, however, Snow appeared to be in good form. He took a lively part in the discussion and agreed to join a new committee being set up to investigate heart disease. As he said goodnight to his friends, he told them how much he was looking forward to starting work on this new project and how confident he was of its success. They were never to see him again.

Snow went to bed at 11.30 still seemingly well, but when he came downstairs the next morning, his housekeeper noticed that he appeared unsteady on his feet. He told her that he felt a little giddy and went to lie down on the sofa, but added that he was sure there was nothing much wrong with him and he would soon be back at work. Indeed not long afterwards he got up and ate a large breakfast before sitting down at his desk to put the finishing touches to his latest project, a manuscript on chloroform. But no sooner had his housekeeper left him when she heard a loud thud and, running back upstairs, found her master on the floor struggling helplessly to get back into his chair. He told her he couldn't understand what was the matter with him: he had never had symptoms like these before. The housekeeper noticed that he appeared to have lost the use of his left arm and leg and that his mouth was twisted to the right. She called for help to lift him on to the sofa and there he stayed for twenty-four hours, neither eating nor sleeping and with a severe pain in his chest, but still insisting that he would soon be better and that he didn't want to trouble anyone.

At six o'clock the next morning he began vomiting blood, and the housekeeper sent for a doctor. By now Snow was paralysed down the entire left side of his body. He remained in this state over the weekend, and then began to slide in and out of delirium. During his lucid moments, he continued to insist that he would soon recover, but on 16 June, a week after he had seemed so well at the medical meeting, his doctors felt that the time had come to tell him that his life was in serious danger. He received the news with the calm with which he had met both good and bad fortune throughout his life, and he died at three o'clock that afternoon, from what had almost certainly been a stroke, with his younger brother, the clergyman Thomas, at his bedside. He was forty-five years old.

Snow's last illness had all the classic signs of chronic renal failure, including his vomiting blood. CRF affects all the other systems of the body and particularly leads to high blood pressure, the main precursor of a stroke. A post-mortem showed that his kidneys were badly diseased and his lungs scarred from the tuberculosis. His years of experiments with toxic gases may have done further unknown damage, and the tiredness and excitability that Joshua Parsons blamed on vegetarianism might have been due to some undiagnosed chronic disease.

John Snow left behind a modest but growing academic reputation. Despite many setbacks and disadvantages, he had lived long enough to achieve some professional success, largely through his anaesthesia practice. His ideas on cholera, though gradually becoming better known, were still widely regarded as bizarre, but his obvious intelligence, diligence and integrity had slowly won him the respect of his colleagues and some measure of recognition. Even so, it had been an austere and solitary existence consisting almost solely of work and study. There are no personal diaries or private letters chronicling great moments of love, anger, success and tragedy, nor even the petty victories and disappointments that mark most people's daily lives. There was no widow or children to mourn him. He had confided to Richardson that he regretted never marrying, and the younger man noticed how at home Snow seemed with Richardson's own family and with those of other friends and, in particular, how much he enjoyed hearing children chattering and laughing around him.

The way in which his work on cholera had been first ignored and then dismissed so relentlessly for so long had been hard to bear even for his stoic nature. He had sometimes talked of his frustration and once expressed the rather bitter view to Richardson that 'nothing so inevitably tends to transform an earnest, inquiring and enthusiastic man into a supercilious, superficial and cold-hearted egotist as translation from the stool of self-reliance and independence into the gilded chair of office'. Richardson said that Snow had not expected an easy passage for his ideas. He realised, of course, that they ran counter to those of many powerful people in both science and politics, and he didn't assume that he would be allowed to go on his way unopposed. 'But he did sometimes expect a more deliberate and considerate attention to his hard-wrought labours than he received and deserved,' Richardson observed.

Struggling to overcome his grief at the loss of the man he had loved and championed, Richardson finished off the task that Snow had been engaged on when he died and saw his last piece of work through to its final publication. He wrote the following in the preface: 'With the fact of my late friend's death not fully realised, with the sensation still on me at intervals – like one who has lost a part of his own body and yet at times conceives the lost present – that he cannot possibly be so far away; I may perchance be pardoned for any deficiencies in style or matter. I have done my best and leave it so.'

As news of Snow's death spread, some of those who had worked with him spoke of their sadness and admiration. Dr Hooper Attree, a former house surgeon at the Middlesex where most of the Broad Street hospital cases had been taken, called on his colleagues to pay some form of public tribute to Snow. 'Who does not remember his frankness, his cordiality, his honesty, the absence of all disguise or affectation under an apparent off-hand manner?' he asked. 'Her Majesty the Queen has been deprived of the future valuable services of a trustworthy, well-deserving, much-esteemed subject. The poor have lost in him a real friend in the hour of need.'

And John French, medical officer at the Poland Street workhouse infirmary for over forty years, had a perceptive comment to make. French had first come across Snow in 1849 when the pair saw a pauper woman through a difficult labour. 'Since the days of Jenner no physician has rendered more important service to mankind than Dr Snow,' he wrote. 'When his doctrine respecting the mode in which cholera is communicated becomes comprehended by Secretaries-of-State and Generals Commanding-in-Chief, then "outbreaks" of cholera – that is, large numbers of persons attacked at once in a district – will become rare events.' French added: 'Although ephemeral criticism has been uniformly against him, yet I venture to predict that the facts brought to light by his indefatigable industry will prove that he was by far the most important investigator of the subject of cholera who has yet appeared.'

Having printed many of Snow's research papers, the *Medical Times and Gazette* gave him a fulsome tribute but the capricious *Lancet* dismissed him in two contemptuous sentences: 'This well-known physician died at his house in Sackville Street from an attack of apoplexy. His researches on chloroform and other anaesthetics were appreciated by the profession.' Cholera wasn't mentioned.

And there for some years the cholera controversy was to remain. As usual once the immediate threat to life had receded, the disease largely dropped off the political agenda, but the need to clean up Britain's disgusting towns and cities did not. The miasmatists continued to bicker with the contagionists; the landlords, the water companies and the 'nuisance' traders fought a fierce but ultimately lost battle against the sanitary reformers; the engineer Joseph Bazalgette started work on London's sewers, and John Snow lay in his grave in London's Brompton Cemetery, largely forgotten except by a small circle of friends and admirers such as Richardson, Edwin Lankester and Joshua Parsons and, now firmly among their number, the Reverend Henry Whitehead.

CHAPTER 16

End Game

The attack was dreadful, threatening the metropolis with desolation, but the early discovery of the channel of distribution and the application of hygiene measures cut it short.

William Farr, Compiler of Abstracts, Office of the Registrar General, 1868

In July 1866, twelve years after the Broad Street outbreak and eight years after John Snow died, Britain's fourth major cholera epidemic in thirty-five years broke out with huge and now familiar savagery along the north bank of the Thames, from the Tower of London eastwards to the Isle of Dogs, in the area known as the Port of London. The disease had again hit the Middle East and Egypt with great ferocity, but took a new route across Europe, invading the Continent from the south through Spain and Gibraltar, and appearing in Marseilles in the summer of 1865. It arrived in England in Southampton that September, but the outbreak there was small and easily contained.

The following spring, the Privy Council in London received telegrams from Liverpool and Birkenhead saying that the disease had broken out among German and Dutch immigrants aboard ships on the river Mersey. Large numbers of immigrants from infected parts of the Continent were arriving at England's eastern ports and travelling across country to Liverpool on their way to

New York. The news caused a great deal of alarm, but the authorities acted fast to isolate the victims and once again disaster was avoided. Sporadic cases were recorded in various parts of England in the first half of that year but there was no large outbreak until suddenly, on 11 July 1866, five people died in London's East End, followed by eleven the following day, and twenty the day after. By the beginning of August, the death rate was over 200 a day.

When the government statistician William Farr went over to the East End to see the situation for himself, he was amused to find that one of his local registrars, a Mr Dunstan, had come up with an ingenious scheme for keeping informants at a healthy distance. 'A chair was in front of his desk and upon attempting to draw it nearer, I found it was tied by a rope and could not be pulled from its place,' Farr said. Dunstan could be forgiven his clumsy and misguided attempts at disease prevention: in one week alone in his tiny area he had registered 141 cholera deaths, and three people came in with more reports during Farr's short visit.

Farr noted:

The mortality is overwhelming in some of the districts. In Poplar 145, and in Bow 188 died last week . . . The people are falling ill every hour; you see them of all ages, children and adults, lying about their beds like people under the influence of a deadly poison, some acutely suffering, nearly all conscious of their fate . . . Here the doctor is drawn in by the husband to see the wife now attacked; there the husband lies in spasms; here is an old woman, seated dead with eyes wide open; there lies a fine four-year-old child, his curly head drooping in death.

It was the same story that had been seen so many times before: on the quayside at Sunderland, the lodging houses of Horsleydown, the killing dormitories of Tooting, the respectable residences of Battersea, the alleys of Soho, and in Liverpool, Exeter, Bristol, Glasgow, Newcastle, and cities, towns and villages the length and breadth of the entire country, on and off for nearly forty years. This time, however, seventeen years after John Snow first published his cholera theory to a nation that refused to listen, his legacy was at last to bear fruit.

As the death toll rose steadily in the East End, the Bishop of London, Archibald Tait, wrote to *The Times* announcing the setting up of a hardship fund. 'No-one can read the reports of the state of the East of London without understanding that there must be a great amount of suffering at this time among the poor,' he said. 'I have information from the clergy, who are labouring with much self-denial and often at the risk of their lives . . . that money is imperatively required.' The next day Catherine Gladstone, wife of the soon-to-be Prime Minister William, wrote asking for donations towards a home for cholera orphans and convalescents. Queen Victoria and the Prince of Wales, perhaps keen to avoid being accused of flaunting their wealth, donated a mere £500 and £200 respectively. The rest of the country, however, felt no such constraints, and an astounding £70,000 flooded in. 'The simple description of some of the scenes I witnessed . . . at once called public attention to the distress and courage of the people,' wrote Farr. 'The fact expressed in the oft-cited sentence "The people of East London want help" was sufficient in England to set hundreds of benevolent people in motion.'

But the bishop had another plea to make; as well as cash, the East End urgently needed more helpers, and he appealed for clergy volunteers, particularly men with previous experience of cholera. Among those to offer his services was Henry Whitehead, still a lowly London curate, and now, since his experiences in Broad Street, a fervent disciple of John Snow. Whitehead had left Soho in 1856 for a church in another Westminster slum, St Matthew's in Great Peter Street, an area whose reputation was best summed up by its local name of Devil's Acre. In 1864, however, the newly married Whitehead joined his former boss, Prebendary Stooks, previously vicar of St Luke's, Berwick Street, at a church in Highgate

Rise, North London. Stooks tried hard to dissuade Whitehead from going to the East End, warning him about the grave risks to his wife and newborn daughter, and giving consent only after Whitehead agreed to pay for a substitute curate out of his own pocket and promised not to return home until the epidemic was safely over. 'It was then that I first made my acquaintance with East London,' Whitehead remembered. 'Until this time, though I had lived in London for 15 years, I had seldom gone eastward of the Aldgate pump.'

Once he did venture past Aldgate and arrived in Bethnal Green, Whitehead found himself in distinguished company. There with their sleeves rolled up in the thick of the suffering were some of the leading members of the Oxford Movement, a group of intellectual clerics who were campaigning for the Church of England to return to its pre-Reformation, Catholic roots, among them Edward Pusey, Regius Professor of Hebrew at Oxford University. Of more immediate interest to Whitehead, however, was a less celebrated member of another profession. John Netten Radcliffe, a Yorkshireman like John Snow, was a forty-year-old doctor from a medical family who had seen more cholera than he cared to think about while serving as a surgeon in the Crimea and had been decorated for his contribution. Now back in England, he was investigating the East End outbreak on behalf of John Simon, medical officer to the Privy Council. Simon had been on Sir Benjamin Hall's Committee for Scientific Inquiry with William Farr and had put his name to the Board of Health's attempt to grab the credit for Snow's 'Grand Experiment'.

One of Radcliffe's tasks was to track down the source of the epidemic, and in this he proved indefatigable. Even though he was recovering from a serious illness, he wandered the streets and courtyards of the East End with Henry Whitehead at his side in a classic 'shoe leather' inquiry. Radcliffe was later to write: 'In carrying out the investigation concerning the earliest cases, I had the good fortune to be assisted by the Reverend H. Whitehead, to whom medicine is in great measure indebted for that elaborate investigation of the cholera outbreak in the parish of St James's which, it is now known, gives to Dr Snow's opinion of its origin a probability practically amounting to a demonstration.' But Whitehead would accept no credit from Radcliffe. 'He has been good enough to say that I rendered him some assistance on this occasion,' he commented. 'But the only assistance he needed was of a kind very easily given, namely the support of my arm whilst he limped about the banks of the river Lea, still suffering from the effects of rheumatic fever.'

Whatever their disagreement about each other's contribution, the doctor and the priest were of one mind about what it was that they were looking for. Doctors and social campaigners were now beginning to accept that polluted water must indeed be a major culprit in the spread of cholera. There had been no great moment of revelation, and Snow's name was seldom mentioned except by a few insiders like Whitehead and Radcliffe; it was simply that the sheer weight of evidence was finally proving overwhelming. Not everyone agreed about the precise nature of the role that water had to play, however, and some hardline miasmatists including Edwin Chadwick and Florence Nightingale were still clinging desperately to their creed.

Government statistician William Farr, whose data on cholera deaths had proved so crucial to John Snow, was a close friend of Florence Nightingale and had long shared her anti-contagionist views. He had once written of a 'disease mist' that hovered in the air over London 'like an angel of death' whenever an epidemic was rife. As a member of Hall's committee back in 1854, he had compared the cholera mortality rates for each London district with the elevation of the area concerned and found that the further a district was from the lowest point in the capital – in other words, from the river Thames – the lower the death rate, the only exception to this being the Broad Street area. Farr and his colleagues had seen this as more evidence that the culprit was bad gas given off by the dirty river.

Farr was six years older than Snow, the son of a dirt-poor Shropshire farm labourer. He had been sent from home at the tender age of eight to learn 'the art and mystery of husbandry', but from this unpromising beginning he had managed to make his way in the world. He had been fortunate enough to be virtually adopted by a wealthy local man who gave the boy a good general education and then paid for him to start medical training. After his benefactor's death Farr had qualified as an apothecary, and developed along the way a special interest and expertise in the newly emerging specialisms of hygiene and medical statistics. In 1839 he found his niche when he was put in charge of statistics at the Registrar General's Office, where he spent the remaining forty years of his career. Civil registration of births, marriages and deaths had become a legal requirement in 1836, partly due to a growing realisation that collecting data on the causes of death would help in the fight against disease, and the Registrar General's Office was set up to administer the scheme.

Farr first came across Nightingale at a London dinner party in the autumn of 1856. He was an unknown government official while she was a national heroine fresh from her triumph in the Crimea, but the pair struck up a close friendship based on their common interest in public health, and soon after meeting they made a pact: he would help with her campaign to improve the health of the army while she would help him with his efforts to do the same for the civilian population. They went on to correspond for nearly twenty years and formed something of a mutual admiration society, Farr at one point writing to express the hope that: 'God grant that you may live long, a martyr truly – a witness – an angel – a messenger – but also an apostle', while she referred to him as her patron saint.

By 1866, however, Farr's miasmatist views, unlike Nightingale's, had begun to change, and on 30 July that year, with the East End outbreak at its height, he wrote to his colleague at the Registrar General's Office, the water analyst Edward Frankland:

On further studying the subject, my suspicions of the East London water are very much strengthened. The weather has been dry, and it is probable that the Lea water has been scanty and the canals and cuts, in a vile state, are in dangerous proximity ... The mortality is terrible just in the area of the East London supply and in other parts slight; it has been so for two weeks and quite reminds me of the Southwark slaughter.

By 'the Southwark slaughter' Farr meant the high death rate on the south bank of the Thames – part of the district covered by John Snow's Grand Experiment – during the epidemics of 1849 and 1854. And in a pattern reminiscent of Southwark, and of Soho too, although Farr didn't say so, the vast majority of the East End deaths were concentrated in a small area; in this case, the affected streets exactly matched those served by the East London Waterworks Company. So while Radcliffe and Whitehead scoured Whitechapel, Poplar and Bethnal Green on the trail of the case that had triggered the outbreak – the 'index' case, like that of baby Lewis in Broad Street – Farr was pursuing an investigation of his own, namely looking for murky secrets at the East London Waterworks.

The East London Waterworks Company had gone into business in 1807 on thirty acres of land in the area known as Old Ford in Bow, taking their water from the river Lea which runs north-south through the East End and joins the Thames just east of the Isle of Dogs. By 1850 the company had moved their intake higher up the river to a place called Lea Bridge, had cut a canal from the Lea across Hackney Marsh to Old Ford, and built six open reservoirs, one at Lea Bridge, one at Stamford Hill and four at Old Ford. Five years later, the company introduced filter beds at Lea Bridge to comply with new legislation. They were still pumping all of their water from the river Lea at Lea Bridge, but while some went direct from there to the northern part of their region, the rest was now carried to Old Ford in an iron pipe, stored in covered reservoirs and then pumped to customers in the southern part of their district. The company's remaining open reservoirs at Old Ford and Stamford Hill had by then been put out of use, or so they insisted.

When Farr published his figures for cholera deaths for the last week in July, he also made public his concerns about East London Water, but unfortunately his description of the company's operations was wrong. 'The canals and the basin [of the Port of London] are full of foul water and are apparently connected with the Limehouse Cut, the Hackney Cut and the River Lea,' he wrote.

> The East London Waterworks canal draws its supply from the river at Lea Bridge where there is a reservoir, and [the canal] runs for a couple of miles by the side of the Hackney Cut down to its other reservoirs north of Bow and near the Lea. The present cholera field derives its waters from these works. It is right to add that the water has hitherto borne a comparison with the other London waters in Professor Frankland's analyses. Today at Poplar the water looks clear and no complaints are made of its quality. The company will no doubt take exemplary pains to filter its waters, but it is not easy to guarantee the purity of water drawn from such a river as the Lea . . .

Farr also called in at the Home Office to warn the then Home Secretary, Spencer Horatio Walpole, about the choice of venue for the forthcoming Whitebait Dinner, an annual gourmet affair held on the Thames and a tradition among senior politicians. 'It appeared singular . . . that while the cholera was raging at Blackwall on the north side of the Thames, it was scarcely felt on the southern shore at Greenwich, although people were freely crossing the river,' Farr recalled. 'A dinner at Blackwall was then a hazardous experiment, while a whitebait dinner at Greenwich was attended with no unusual risk.'

The East London Waterworks Company wasted no time in responding to the criticisms. No sooner had the ink dried on Farr's accusations than the company's chief engineer, Charles Greaves, stormed into his office complaining that 'the implied charge against the company was ill founded and the description of the works incorrect'. Farr showed him the information he was working from and when Greaves pointed out that his maps were out of date, Farr told the engineer that if the company produced a correct version, he, Farr, would forward it to the newspapers that same day. Greaves promised to do so but instead wrote to the press himself. In this he was motivated not by the interests of the company but by a sense of public duty, he explained.

'I observe in the weekly return of the Registrar General, a statement so injurious to the East London Waterworks Company and so likely to create public alarm that, although I might on the company's behalf have been prepared to remain silent, I think you will feel me justified in asking a place in your columns for the purpose of allaying what I fear may be greatly misapprehended and may, if unexplained, cause considerable public alarm,' ran his letter in the next day's issue of *The Times*. From Farr's statement, Greaves said, every reader would, first, assume that the company's water ran in an open canal, dangerously close to a source of pollution, and, second, would conclude that while the company might claim to filter their water, they were in reality supplying it unfiltered.

The truth, said Greaves, was that the water was carried in pipes and 'never saw the light of day' on its entire journey between the filter bed and the consumer. 'The canal alluded to by the Registrar, having been since 1853 disused for all purposes of supply, is only maintained as a drain from the filter to a lower part of the river,' Greaves pointed out, adding that 'not a drop of unfiltered water has for several years past been supplied by the company for any purpose'. And while Farr had admitted that the East London Company's water had 'hitherto borne a comparison with the other London waters' and that 'today the water looks clear and no complaints are made of its quality', these statements were, said Greaves, to quote a phrase, 'in dangerous proximity' to the other, erroneous, parts of the report.

I impute no intentional misrepresentation and I make no complaint [he went on], although when I found on calling this afternoon at the Registrar General's office that he was using and acting upon an obsolete map of this district I felt that better information should be in use by so important an officer, and that if it had been so, the East London Waterworks Company would have escaped an unmerited censure, and the public mind an unfounded cause of alarm.

The next day Farr paid a return visit to Greaves at Old Ford, where he found the engineer by now 'deeply impressed with the serious nature of the inquiry', and it was while Farr was being shown around the site that he learnt something that gave him a clue as to what might have gone wrong. Returning to his office he ordered Professor Frankland's assistant, Mr Valentin, back from his summer holiday in Ramsgate and then packed the unfortunate official off to the East End, notebook in hand.

Farr had discovered that while the company insisted that their old, uncovered reservoirs were never used, they remained connected to the covered reservoirs at Old Ford, so it was still technically possible to draw water from them. And, what was more, running between the two sets of reservoirs was the river Lea 'in a most filthy state'. The statistician had also noticed something else quite remarkable: all the deaths were in the area supplied from Old Ford; the region that received its water direct from Lea Bridge was cholera-free. He told Valentin: 'Go to Mr Greaves, whom you will find at Old Ford, and get him to allow you to take waters for analysis from his covered reservoir at Old Ford, from the two reservoirs uncovered, and from the Lea Bridge, where you can get the water before and after filtration.'

On his arrival at Old Ford, Valentin was met by Greaves and also by a Mr Maine, the man in charge at Lea Bridge who happened to mention in passing that he had recently eaten some excellent eels out of the Old Ford reservoir. Valentin passed this anecdote on to his boss. A few days later the *East End News* published some curious letters from some of East London Waterworks' customers. One, from a Mr Furgusson of Bow Lane, was headed: 'Can an Eel Pass Through a Filter Bed?' 'The second week of June last, our water pipe was stopped up, and as I am a plumber I cut the pipe, and to my astonishment found a dead eel, nine inches in length, which must have come through the above works and which is quite demonstrative that the water is not filtered; so if you think this hint will be the means of the company improving the filtering, you will greatly oblige me by giving this publicity,' Furgusson wrote.

And Alexander Russell of the almost certainly inappropriately named Paradise Cottages, also in Bow, had a similar story to tell: 'A short time since the water supply to my residence was stopped, from what cause I could not imagine, and I was without a supply five days. At length I took off the tap and to my astonishment found an eel, 14 inches in length. It was in a putrid state and the stench arising from it was most fearful.' Mr Russell had just lost two of his children to cholera, he added. The following week, two fire hydrants were opened in Commercial Road, Whitechapel, and 'at least a bushel' (probably equivalent to about a large basketful) of mussels poured out. The only way that the shellfish could have reached the hydrants was via the pipes of the East London Waterworks Company.

Notices quickly went up throughout the East End warning people to boil their drinking water, while back in Henry Whitehead's old patch they were taking no chances; the sanitary committee of St James's Westminster chained up the handle of every pump in the parish. And like Whitehead in Soho, William Farr was struck by a widespread misunderstanding among members of the public when it came to drinking water. When he commiserated with a newly bereaved widower in Poplar, for example, the man told him, 'We never drank water, neither my wife nor myself.' 'What do you drink then?' Farr asked. 'Beer and a tumbler of spirits and water at night.' 'Hot water?' 'No, cold.'

Meanwhile as Valentin busied himself around the waterworks collecting samples for Professor Frankland, and Farr and Greaves squabbled over canals and reservoirs, so John Netten Radcliffe and Henry Whitehead were following up leads in their attempt to uncover the index case. There had been a few deaths in May in different parts of London from what was described as 'choleraic diarrhoea' and 'simple diarrhoea', but only one death registered as Asiatic cholera, and that was in south London, six weeks before the East End outbreak. Two little girls had also died of cholera on 25 June, two weeks before the disease exploded, but they lived over fives miles away. Finally, Radcliffe and Whitehead tracked down what the doctor concluded was 'the earliest unquestionable case' in East London. On 26 June, a couple called Hedges who worked at a brush-making factory near Bow Bridge went down with Asiatic cholera and died the next day. Both had been in excellent health and both were struck down at exactly the same time with no warning, 'as though they had swallowed a poisonous dose', Radcliffe said.

The Hedges lived in Priory Street, Bromley by Bow, on the banks of the river Lea, which was at that time on the eastern-most edge of the metropolis. Radcliffe described their cottage as 'a small, wretched four-room dwelling', but added that it was neither smaller nor more wretched than scores of others in the area, and as far as ventilation and the open space behind it were concerned, it was 'infinitely better circumstanced than hundreds of houses of no better class within cannon shot'. At the back of the house was a small outbuilding with a water closet that had to be flushed by hand, the drain from which ran under the house and connected with a sewer that discharged into the river Lea at Bow Bridge, half a mile below the Old Ford reservoirs. By 1866, Joseph Bazalgette's great main drainage system was well under construction, but the work was still not finished in East London.

Radcliffe and Whitehead made the most extensive inquiries into the Hedges' habits and into how they had spent the days leading up to their deaths but, like John Snow with the servant at Albion Terrace, they eventually had to confess themselves at a complete loss to explain how the couple had contracted the disease. Certainly anyone who still believed that dissolute living had a part to play found nothing to support their theory here: the Hedges

were the very models of respectability. 'They were persons of regular and temperate habits, in excellent repute with their employer,
their work fellows and their neighbours,' reported Radcliffe, and
during the two weeks before their deaths they had followed their
usual domestic routine. On the previous Sunday they walked with
one of their daughters and a friend through Poplar and the Isle of
Dogs, took the ferry over to Greenwich and strolled in Greenwich
Park. On their way home, the four shared one pint of beer between
them at an ale house near the park gates. That day the couple, their
three children and the friend had rabbit pie and potatoes for dinner,
and the family finished up the left-overs the next day. Apart from
the pie, the Hedges' diet consisted of their usual tea or coffee and
bread and butter. On Monday, the day before they were taken ill,
the couple spent the evening with a friend at a travelling circus in
Stratford.

As far as any one could tell, neither Hedges nor his wife had
been in contact with anyone who had just arrived from an infected
part of the Continent. None of their children nor the friends with
whom they had spent their last days suffered the slightest illness.
Not one of the 200 men, women and children who worked at the
brush factory had had bowel complaints of any kind, and Radcliffe
found no suspicious cases of sickness among any of the neighbours
at the time that Mr and Mrs Hedges were struck down, although
the doctor did comment that it was hard to be sure of accurate
information in such a densely populated district where people were
constantly coming and going.

'Their cases were punched, so to speak, as clearly and definely
out of the population as a hole is punched out of a tissue,' Radcliffe
wrote.

The commencing activity of the choleraic poison in Bromley on
26 June must be looked upon, so far as our present knowledge of
the facts extend, as a phenomenon entirely independent of the
ordinary summer diarrhoea and cholera of this climate . . . How
the poison originated or . . . where the individuals of the resident

population earliest attacked first contracted the disease and in what manner, the known facts do not show. In the case of Hedges and his wife, this knowledge died with them, but the presumption is that they contracted the disease – or more correctly perhaps swallowed the poison – at the same time and under the same circumstances to which they alone of their family, their fellow workers or their neighbours were at that time exposed.

But by whatever means the Hedges had contracted cholera, the route by which they passed it on to people living right across the East End of London was steadily being exposed. In their search for the index case, Radcliffe and Whitehead also uncovered more circumstantial evidence against East London Waterworks to add to Farr's dossier. There had been a tiny outbreak in the parish of East Ham in mid-July, for example, which proved 'exceedingly fatal in certain most wretched of cottages known as King Harry Row, Sun Row East and Sun Row West,' Radcliffe reported. 'Now the East London Water Company's supply from Old Ford extends into East Ham at one point only and here it is distributed solely to two separate houses, the Rising Sun Inn and Potato Hall, and two rows of cottages. Those cottages are those known as King Harry Row and Sun Row East. The inhabitants of Sun Row West also freely use the water as the only dependable source of supply within reach.'

And in August, when the Whitechapel medical officer, Mr Liddle, ordered a house-to-house inspection of his patch, he found a strange anomaly. Among the 2,000 residents of Petticoat Lane, home to the now famous street market, there were just four cases of diarrhoea. On the same day in the surrounding streets, however, there were 245 cases of diarrhoea, fourteen cases of 'choleraic diarrhoea', one case of 'diarrhoea passing into cholera' and twenty-two cases of cholera. Petticoat Lane obtained its water from the New River Company. The other streets were supplied by the East London Water Company from Old Ford. 'On one side of a line defined only by a difference of water supply, the conditions of the population as to comfort and hygienic state being in all other respects analogous, there was found an epidemic actively prevailing, and, on the other, hardly an indication of its existence,' said Radcliffe.

But another veteran of the Committee for Scientific Inquiry, the meteorologist and ballooning adventurer James Glaisher, was still convinced that the origins of epidemic disease lay within his own specialism and he had a different theory to offer. Glaisher was much intrigued by the appearance of a blue mist, first reported the week the outbreak began and last seen during the previous epidemic. 'It has extended from Aberdeen to the Isle of Wight and is of the same tint of blue everywhere,' he reported. 'I do not know the nature of this blue influence, but the fact of its presence not having been noticed since the cholera period of 1854 until now points out a possible connection.' Radcliffe, however, was unimpressed by the theory of the blue peril. 'Neither the meteorology of the period, nor the altitude nor the nature of the soil nor the density of population nor filth nor the state of the sewerage nor locality, affords any explanation of the peculiar locations of the outbreak in the East London districts,' he concluded. 'There is but one condition known which might become capable of propagating cholera common to the whole area of the outbreak, namely the water supply.'

William Farr, meanwhile, was more certain than ever, not only that the blame lay with the East London Waterworks but that it had something to do with the reservoirs at Old Ford. Professor Frankland's tests on Valentin's samples showed that on 9 August, one month into the outbreak, the water in the covered reservoir was actually dirtier than that in the open reservoirs, and Farr now suspected that earlier that summer the company had secretly taken water from its supposedly disused open reservoirs and that those reservoirs had somehow been contaminated with 'cholera poison'.

On one of his several visits to the area, the statistician described a deceptively attractive scene:

I went by the Great Eastern Railway from the Shoreditch Station to Lea Bridge, passing close by the open reservoirs which looked as placidly in the light as if they had never held poison that killed thousands . . . Gnats were playing over the waters, and the swallows, in active pursuit, clustered over a particular reservoir that appeared to afford them especially good sport. The workmen were wheeling away barrows full of gravel or sand. The great engine was at work. The waters lie in the midst of rich meadows on which many cows were feeding, and are surrounded by an amphitheatre of houses and churches, crowned to the north with the Alexandra Palace.

The river Lea itself was high at that point with what appeared to be fresh, fast-running water. Farr walked over the low, spongy fields and then took a carriage northwards to Walthamstow where he called on the local registrar, a surgeon called Browne, 'in his comfortable house'. There had been no cholera deaths in this area in any previous epidemic and none in this, Browne told him, and many of the newest and best houses in the district were supplied by the East London Waterworks. 'The further inspection confirmed the conviction that the cholera stuff was not distributed in the waters supplied from Lea Bridge and that, on the whole, the waters of the Lea at that point are not impurer to any appreciable extent than those of the Thames,' Farr decided.

Farr now told Greaves that he had 'by the sheer force of circumstantial evidence come definitively to the conclusion that the company had used the open reservoirs for a certain time up to the outbreak of the cholera'. He had an offer to make: 'If he would of his own knowledge affirm that they had not been used, I would engage to say that the Registrar General would publish his letter and that I for one would accept his statement as conclusively true.' Greaves himself gave no reply, but the company put out a statement claiming that their staff at Old Ford were ready, without exception, to swear on oath that the connection between the covered and the open reservoirs hadn't been opened for at least two years.

By now, however, despite their bravado, Charles Greaves and the East London Waterworks Company were fighting a losing battle, and gradually, inch by inch, the truth was dragged out of them. After having admitted that, contrary to official records, it was still possible to use the open reservoirs, Greaves then went a step further and told Professor Frankland that although 'communication can be established between these reservoirs and the pumping wells supplying the public, it was never done except in the case of emergency'. Later that year, the Pollution of Rivers Commission looked into the affair and in his evidence to this body, Greaves, in Farr's words, 'advanced another step' and revealed that 'a small quantity' of water was taken out of one of the open reservoirs that year. He didn't know the date; it was probably June, but he couldn't say definitely.

The full sorry tale was eventually unearthed by a Board of Trade inspector, one Captain William Tyler of the Royal Engineers. Tyler was called in when a group of East London Waterworks' customers – urged on by Henry Whitehead's temporary boss at Bethnal Green, the rector Septimus Hansard – made an official complaint about their water supply. Tyler learned that the company's works foreman had died suddenly early in 1866 and Greaves had duly appointed a replacement. The engineer said that when he gave the new foreman his instructions, he mentioned the possibility of drawing on the open reservoirs as something to bear in mind, should the water in the covered reservoirs drop so low as to put the pump engine under too great a strain. 'So I suppose he may have acted in that sense,' Greaves said. For his part, the foreman explained that he regarded the open reservoirs as being available for use in just such an emergency. He kept no notes, but he believed he had drawn water from the open reservoir not more than three times that year: at the end of March, at the end of June and some time in early July. He had had no fear of it doing any harm.

It then emerged that the company actually employed a carpenter whose job it was to operate the sluice between the open and covered reservoirs at Old Ford. He had been with East London Waterworks for twenty-four years and did other jobs, but the sluice was his special responsibility. He had opened it frequently during 1864 and 1865, he told Tyler, and three times in 1866. In March that year he had been in the engine house when the engine began to suck in air, and Greaves ordered him to open the sluice. He had left it open for two hours. In June he was in the yard when the engine driver called to him to 'let him have some water', and the foreman ordered him to comply. Then one afternoon in early July – just days after the Hedges died – he had once again allowed stagnant, unfiltered water to run into the covered reservoir.

'When this statement is compared with Mr Greaves' letter and when it is borne in mind that these dependent men were not giving evidence on oath, that the opening of the sluice would be precisely one of those acts of which no record was desired, we can scarcely expect a more explicit statement,' remarked Farr. 'It is enough to have in evidence that immediately before the outbreak in July the foul water of the reservoirs was pumped over parts of East London.' And, according to Frankland, even with the sluice closed, foul water from the most polluted part of the river Lea was still capable of finding its way into the covered reservoirs. 'When the tide [of the nearby river Lea] was high and the water of the reservoir was low, the permeation of the water through the gravely bottom into the reservoir was, by hydraulic principle, inevitable.'

Captain Tyler decided to put this to the test. Over one weekend, then, East London Waterworks duly pumped out an entire reservoir to within a foot of the bottom, and Tyler spent his Sunday afternoon wading about in the water. He found dirty water spurting in across the old sluice and through several of the roof supports, as well as clear signs of heavy soaking through the brickwork sides and at the foot where brick met gravel. 'There were also, as it were, springs issuing below the level of the surface which became more visible as the water decreased in depth,' Tyler said, 'and it was impossible to avoid the conclusion that if more of the bottom could have been laid bare, more of these issues would have been seen and a greater quantity of water would have been found to enter the reservoir.' In fact, it proved impossible to empty the reservoir completely. 'The water came in faster than it could be pumped out by a powerful engine,' recounted Farr. 'The patience of the waiting company was exhausted: the water still came in. Cholera flux, with the other excremental matters in the channel of the Lea, thus must have found its way from the reservoirs to the pump well of the company at Old Ford.'

The Lea at Old Ford was far dirtier that summer than it had been during the previous cholera outbreak in 1854, for since 1861 the sewers not only of the East End of London but of the entire districts of Stratford and West Ham on the Essex side had been flushed into the river, and twice a day the tide washed this filth up and down stream, close to the site of the Old Ford reservoirs. In his evidence to the Rivers Commission, a Mr Marshall, a government sanitary engineer based at West Ham, described how every low tide exposed a large part of the river bank covered with slimey mud that looked foul and smelt worse. 'In hot weather, what kind of sensation have you when walking near that mud?' asked one of the commissioners. 'I always have the sensation that I should like to be somewhere else,' replied Marshall.

It was against this background that one day in early July 1866, probably the 9th or 10th, at two o'clock in the afternoon, according to Farr, 'when the covered reservoir was at the lowest ebb, and the dregs of the water were drawn ... the pumps gave unmistakable signs of distress; the engine driver called out for water and then told carpenter to open the sluice and let in the contents of the northern, stagnant pond ... How often this was repeated in July it is impossible to tell,' Farr went on, 'But if the supply from Lea Bridge in July was less than in May, the East London Company must have drawn on its open reservoirs, for in their return they give the quantities supplied at 2,167,885 gallons a day more in July than in May. They distributed 636 million gallons in July. Where did it all come from?' The question was, by then, rhetorical.

The East End epidemic lasted for three months, and over 4,000 East Enders lost their lives. While real progress had at last been made in understanding how cholera spread, little had changed in terms of treatment. Most of the East End hospital cases went to the London in Whitechapel – the 'orspital, as it was locally known – where the doctors tried all manner of new remedies in the forlorn hope of finding something that might work.

Dr Fraser, for example, tried steam inhalation and, finding it useless, moved on to large, two-hourly doses of castor oil, but this proved so unpleasant that his patients rebelled and refused to take it. He next turned his attention to a currently fashionable remedy known as the 'Rubini', presumably after its inventor who seems to have passed into obscurity. This consisted of a highly concentrated solution of camphor in alcohol, given in doses of five to twenty minims (5–20 drops) on sugar or in water every five minutes. However, the resulting gluey mixture had the effect of clogging up the patients' mouth and making them retch. One victim, in a severe state of collapse, was only prevented from choking to death by the prompt action of an attendant who scooped the stuff out of his mouth with a spoon handle. 'The patients in several instances begged that its use might be discontinued on account of the distress which it occasioned,' reported the *Lancet*. 'In some cases it was tried every quarter or half hour, but always with the same result: the camphor being rejected by vomiting.'

One of Fraser's colleagues, Dr Clark, tried a combination of castor oil and 'saline lemonade' to no avail, and Dr Davies had no more success with a grain of podophyllin (a plant extract, now used to treat genital warts) and camphor, alternating every hour with sulphuric acid and cyanide. The London team also tried injecting opium into very sick patients, but all of them died. And matters went no better at other hospitals. At Guy's, across the Thames in south-east London, for example, Dr Owen Rees reportedly poured 'gallons' of nitrous oxide gas into two patients but 'the proceeding was not attended with any success', while in Southampton, where a few cases had broken out again that summer, surgeons Griffin and Bencraft carried out a long but ineffective trial with ice-bags to the spine, and other doctors were forced to give up on arsenic and subcutaneous injections of turpentine.

The work to track down those responsible for the East End deaths, however, was meeting with greater success, and Captain Tyler was soon reporting back to Whitehall that the truth 'had finally been admitted by the officers and servants of the company'. The use of unfiltered water stored in an uncovered reservoir was 'indefensible', he added, 'and a distinct infringement of the provisions of the Metropolis Water Supply Act of 1852'. The Board of Trade duly wrote to the directors of East London Waterworks Company telling them that the residents' complaint against them had been upheld and that they were 'required within a reasonable time to remove the grounds of such complaint'. The directors declared themselves ready to comply but at the same time they had a complaint of their own to make, namely that the conscientious Captain Tyler had exceeded his powers as a Board of Trade official. The directors might have thought themselves lucky. The maximum penalty that the law prescribed for a company supplying contaminated drinking water was a fine of £200. For killing over 4,000 of their customers and lying about it, there were no sanctions available.

'The public is hitherto very imperfectly protected against certain extreme dangers which the malfeasance of a water company supplying, perhaps, half a million customers may suddenly bring upon great masses of population,' wrote John Simon. 'Its colossal power of life and death is something for which till recently there has been no precedent in the history of the world.' And describing the £200 penalty as 'utterly incommensurate with the magnitude of the public danger', Simon said that when the law was introduced in 1852, 'The state of science did not yet enable the Legislature to know, as it must now know, that a water company distributing sewage-tainted water may, in a day, take hundreds of lives.'

Not everyone took the lesson to heart. The following year, 1867, John Netten Radcliffe was called in to investigate the serially offending Southwark and Vauxhall Company, whose drinking water was said to resemble 'diluted pea soup or a yellow November fog', and whose supply to Bermondsey public baths was 'frequently quite useless', even though the company had put a strainer over its supply pipe 'to keep back dead fish and other matters'.

But with the exposure of the East London Waterworks Company came the final vindication for John Snow. The case for cholera being spread from the sick to the healthy primarily through contaminated drinking water was now proved beyond the doubts of any but a few fanatical and now completely marginalised miasmatists. The *Lancet* commented: 'The lesson ... for the public to learn from that experience of cholera in regard to the supply of water is too obvious to admit of a moment's doubt.'

John Simon, who like William Farr had been a miasmatist for his entire career, described the discovery of the connection between polluted water and epidemic disease as the most outstanding medical achievement for a quarter of a century. The same man who, in 1856, had replicated Snow's 'Grand Experiment' and published it under his own name and that of the Board of Health, wrote in his annual report:

> In the autumn of 1849, at the height of our terrible second epidemic, Dr John Snow, in an admirably lucid and original little paper ... advanced the doctrine ... that cholera propagates itself from person to person by means of the intestinal discharges of the sick, and he claimed ... that it gave the true explanation of the influence which sewage-polluted water had been seen to exercise ... Dr Snow in 1849 was not able to furnish proofs of his doctrine against which, at first sight, some strong arguments seemed to hold; but afterwards distinct experiments, as well as much new collateral information established as almost certain that his bold conjecture had been substantially right.

Simon went on to refer to Broad Street and the Grand Experiment and although he then quoted at length from his own 1856 publication, belated amends, of a sort, had nevertheless been made.

Never again was Britain to be at the mercy of a great cholera epidemic, although isolated cases of the disease continued to break out here and there for the next twenty years. In 1875 Joseph Bazalgette's magnificent main drainage system for London was finally completed. Gradually other towns and cities were provided with decent sewers, and drinking water became both clean and plentiful. In 1892, sixty years after cholera had made its first journey across the North Sea, the disease was on the move once more, revisiting all of its favourite haunts such as Mecca, Jeddah, Baghdad, Constantinople, Moscow and St Petersburg. At the end of August, it reached Hamburg yet again, and the British government swung into now familiar action, sending doctors to oversee precautions on the coasts, and issuing advice about prevention and containment. The medical officer for the Port of London took himself off to Gravesend to inspect vessels entering the Thames, while the authorities at Hull, Grimsby, Liverpool and Southampton began isolating or refusing entry to newly arrived passengers and setting up floating hospitals.

'I left Hamburg a few days ago and the cholera had then appeared there,' reported a *Times* correspondent. 'It is now raging in that place with a violence that threatens a mortality that will outstrip the record of Astrakhan.' Between 7,000 and 8,000 people died that month in the German port, where conditions were so poor that sewage ran out of the houses and then back in again in the form of drinking water 'after a little tour in the foul river and even fouler waterworks', *The Times* said. Britain, in the meantime, stood poised once more to face the approaching disaster. It never came. By the end of the century, the government had classified cholera as a rare and exotic disease.

In the autumn of 1883, seventeen years after the East End outbreak, the world heard that the German scientist Robert Koch had identified the minute, comma-shaped bacterium – the *Vibrio cholerae* – responsible for the disease known as cholera in human beings, and established beyond doubt that it was spread mainly by means of contaminated drinking water, but could also be transmitted in food and, occasionally, on soiled linen.

In fact, as early as 1854 – the very year of the Broad Street out-break – an Italian scientist named Filippo Pacini had made the discovery for which Koch was later credited but, much as with the work of John Snow, at the time no one appreciated the significance of his findings.

Vibrii (a type of bacterium that appear to vibrate as they move) are one of the most common organisms to be found in surface water across the globe, and the *Vibrio cholerae* – the cause of the disease – lives in the environment in brackish rivers and coastal waters. Occasional cases of cholera caused by eating raw shellfish have been recorded.

The *Vibrio cholerae* can live for up to five days in foodstuff such as meat, milk and cheese, and for up to two weeks in water. Infected water, once deprived of its source of contamination, then, becomes cholera-free after ten to fourteen days. This, it was thought, explains an epidemic's habit of stopping as suddenly and as unpredictably as it started. However, some new research sug-gests that the bacteria are killed off by what is known as a Vibrio phage – a virus that lives in bacteria. During an epidemic, the theory runs, the phage multiply in the patient's gut and are then excreted along with the bacteria. As the epidemic progresses, the phage build up in the water supply in overwhelming numbers and eventually kill off the bacteria.

When the *Vibrio cholerae* enter the human gut, they multiply very quickly in huge numbers and produce a toxin that acts on the lining of the intestine, turning the cells into virtual 'pumps' that take water and essential salts from the blood and tissues. This fluid is then expelled in the form of litre after litre of watery diarrhoea, along with massive numbers of vibrios that will go on to cause a huge and immediate outbreak if they find their way into the water supply. The 'rice-water' appearance of the diarrhoea is due to a mucus secreted by the gut cells.

All of the terrifying later symptoms – the cramps and spasms, the 'dark blue' body, the sunken eyes, wizened features and corrugated skin that lead to the final total collapse – are in fact secondary symptoms, caused not directly by the bacterium itself but by a massive loss of body fluid. And the thick, black 'tarry' substance found in the victims' veins that led many medical men to conclude that cholera was a disease of the blood is, as John Snow had realised, another result of fluid loss. Death, then, comes from dehydration.

Not everyone reacts to the *Vibrio cholerae* in the same way. Some people have no noticeable symptoms at all, some experience mild diarrhoea while others develop the life-threatening disease that is now known simply as cholera. The reasons for this are not understood, any more than the reasons why different individuals react differently to other pathogens are understood. Previous exposure to the vibrio certainly has a part to play in giving immunity. And people who carry the cystic fibrosis gene are immune from severe attacks because their bodies are less prone to lose fluid. As a result, there is a higher incidence of cystic fibrosis in areas where cholera used to be common: the carriers have survived in greater numbers than the non-carriers. Blood type is also important: those in the commonest group – type O – are the most susceptible to cholera, while those with the rare type AB have about a six-fold lower risk.

A normal, healthy adult must swallow about one million *Vibrio cholerae* in order to be at risk from the disease although, as with all diseases, those who are malnourished or whose immune system is weak for some other reason are more susceptible. And in the case of cholera, people with low levels of gastric acid – for example because they are taking antacids for stomach problems – are also in more danger.

From the beginning of the twentieth century to the 1960s, cholera was confined to South Asia. Then in 1961, a new strain called El Tor emerged to cause a major epidemic in Indonesia and then a global pandemic that has spread across Asia, the Middle East, Africa, South and Central America – and, more recently, parts of Europe. In 1982, however, the 'classic' strain responsible for the nineteenth-century pandemics resurfaced in Bangladesh, rapidly replacing El Tor. Then in 1992, a totally new strain known as *Vibrio cholerae* 0139 was found in India and Bangladesh. The 0139 has not, so far, moved beyond South Asia.

The main emphasis in combating cholera today is still on prevention through clean drinking water and efficient drains and sewers, and the threat of an outbreak in those areas where cholera is endemic is always a major concern whenever wars or natural disasters damage water supplies and sewerage systems, or force people to flee their homes for the primitive conditions of a refugee camp. Until fifty years ago, cholera remained endemic at low levels in parts of Europe, resulting in small isolated outbreaks from time to time. This type of low-level presence can then explode given the right conditions, as it did in Broad Street for example. Until recently the only vaccine available was not very effective, but some new oral vaccines are proving useful.

Treating cholera is simply a matter of replacing as fast as possible the fluid and salts that the body has lost. If the dehydration is not too severe, this is done by giving the patient oral rehydration solution (ORS): simple but scientifically developed drinks of sugar, water and salt. Very sick patients are given these fluids intravenously. In this way victims hovering on the brink of death can be brought almost instantly back to health as if by a miracle.

Some nineteenth-century doctors did recommend giving patients large quantities of water, with or without salt, most notably William Stevens, who claimed great success for what he called the saline treatment. Not everyone had good results with this, however, because much depends on the quantity and constituents of the fluid, and the method and speed with which it is administered. Stevens pestered John Ayrton Paris about the matter to such an extent that the president of the Royal College of Physicians eventually had him thrown out of his office.

So for decades medical men fought over the supposed merits of different poisonous concoctions, subjecting their dying patients to all manner of dreadful and pointless tortures – yet the tragic irony is that all the time a simple cure lay well within their abilities and resources, if only they had understood enough about the action of the disease to use that cure properly. Equally ironic is that our sophisticated twenty-first-century antibiotics and other complex drugs are virtually useless when confronted with the deadly virulence of the *Vibrio cholerae*.

EPILOGUE

With the final end to Britain's cholera epidemics, the main characters in the story went their different ways. After the St James's Vestry inquiry, the Soho doctor Edwin Lankester, who had led the investigation, went on to become the parish medical officer where he proved tireless in his fight against insanitary conditions, much to the annoyance of the local property owners and businessmen. In 1866, the year of the East End outbreak, he published a small book called *Cholera: What it is and how to prevent it*, in which he wrote of that famous night of 7 September 1854, when Snow went before the Board of Guardians: 'He [Snow] was admitted and gave it as his opinion that the pump in Broad Street and that pump alone, was the cause of all the pestilence. He was not believed – not a member of his own profession, not an individual in the parish, believed that Snow was right.'

The hero of the food adulteration scandal, Arthur Hill Hassall, continued his microscopy work to the end of his days. In his autobiography *The Narrative of a Busy Life*, published in 1893, he wrote of his investigations for the Committee for Scientific Inquiry: 'There is not the smallest doubt that the cholera bacillus was present in the discharges in nearly every case and was first seen by me during the cholera epidemic of 1854.' Sadly for Hassall, it had been left to the German doctor Robert Koch some thirty years later to explain just what it was he had been looking at.

William Budd's reputation recovered from the 1849 fungus debacle when he and his Bristol colleagues were discredited after claiming to have discovered the cholera-causing agent, and Budd is now celebrated for his work on another largely water-borne intestinal disease, typhoid.

In July 1855, after just a year at the Board of Health, Sir Benjamin Hall was made Chief Commissioner of Works where he negotiated with the engineer Joseph Bazalgette over the plans for London's sewers. Hall also oversaw the completion of the new Palace of Westminster where Big Ben, the great bell in the clock-tower, bears his nickname.

After twenty years as a curate in the capital, Henry Whitehead left London in 1874 and ended his days as a vicar in rural Cumberland where he threw himself with characteristic energy into local affairs. He kept a portrait of John Snow on his study wall to his dying day to remind him, he said, 'that in any profession, the highest order of work is achieved not by fussy demand "for something to be done" but by patient study of the eternal laws.'

Edwin Chadwick went to his grave holding fast to the miasma theory although, like Florence Nightingale, he lived to see the French chemist Louis Pasteur discover the link between bacteria and disease, and other scientists isolate specific disease-causing organisms. As late as 1890, the year he died, Chadwick was advocating pumping down warmed, fresh air from tall structures like the Eiffel Tower in order to dispel disease.

And five years after Pasteur's breakthrough, Florence Nightingale wrote: 'What does contagion mean? It implies communication of disease from person to person contact. It presupposes the existence of certain germs like the sporules of fungi, which can be bottled up and conveyed any distance attached to clothing, to merchandise . . . There is no end to the absurdities connected with this doctrine. Suffice it to say that in the ordinary sense of the word, there is no proof such as would be admitted in any scientific enquiry that there is any such thing as contagion.'

John Snow is commemorated in Brompton Cemetery by a hand-some memorial paid for by colleagues and admirers, and also in Broadwick Street – as Broad Street is now known – by a pub named after him, a strange tribute to a man who campaigned all his life against alcohol. There is also a replica of the famous pump in the street, although not on the exact site. Over the years Snow's reputation in epidemiology and in anaesthesia has flourished, and he is now regarded as a pioneering figure in both fields. Extraordinary progress has been made in epidemiology since his death, going far beyond the field of communicable disease with which he was concerned into, for example, the links between lung cancer and smoking and between cervical cancer and the Human Papilloma virus, and increasingly into non-medical areas such as social issues. At the US Centers for Disease Control and Prevention (CDC) in Atlanta, Georgia, ground-breaking achievements include steps towards the eradication of smallpox, the identification of the Ebola virus and the tracking down of the causes of Legionnaires disease. When CDC staff are looking for a straightforward solution to an epidemiological problem they are sometimes heard to ask: 'Where is the handle on this pump?'

At his farewell dinner on leaving London, Henry Whitehead recalled some words of John Snow: '"You and I," he would say to me, "may not live to see the day, and my name may be forgotten when it comes, but the time will arrive when great outbreaks of cholera will be things of the past; and it is the knowledge of the way in which the disease is propagated which will cause them to disappear".' In a career distinguished by remarkably accurate insights, on one point at least – that his name would be forgotten – John Snow was eventually to be proved wrong.

AFTERWORD

While scientists argue about the causes of global warming, no one doubts that the earth is getting hotter. According to the World Health Organization, world temperature has gone up by about 0.4°C since the 1970s and is predicted to rise by several degrees more this century.

The implications for human health are immense. There will undoubtedly be some gains, such as a drop in winter deaths in temperate countries, but overall the impact of climate change is likely to be adverse and to include an increased risk from some infectious diseases. Infections carried by mosquitoes and other insects, such as malaria and yellow fever, for example, could become more prevalent if warmer temperatures allow those insects to establish themselves over a wider area.

And there is reason to be concerned about cholera. Along with global warming comes an increase in severe weather events that increase the risk of disease. Floods can cause sewers and wastewater treatment plants to overflow, contaminating surface water and wells, while droughts bring with them the poor sanitary conditions in which cholera, for example, flourishes. And while not directly related, outbreaks of cholera seem to be somehow associated with the climatic event known as El Niño, which has been increasing in frequency over the last thirty years. Some experts believe that El Niño triggered the resurgence of cholera in Peru in 1991, for example.

Recently, some studies have suggested a symbiotic link between the *Vibrio cholerae* and plankton, the tiny organisms that drift in great numbers in fresh or salt water. A rise in sea surface temperatures could cause an increase in plankton and thus in *Vibrio cholerae* and, in turn, in cases of cholera. And some theories predict an increase in the toxicity of *Vibrio cholerae,* again as a result of sea changes related to climate change.

This is a complex issue involving many factors whose combined effects are hugely difficult to predict. It is vital that we attempt to make those predictions, however, and scientists are currently devising models to try to work out the likely impact of global change on the future behaviour of diseases such as cholera. How we cope with any new threat depends on how good their calculations prove to be.

MAIN SOURCES

GENERAL SOURCES

Numerous contemporary issues of the *Lancet* and *The Times*.

Privy Council and Parliamentary Papers in the Public Record Office and Guildhall Library.

Longmate N. *King Cholera*. London: Hamilton, 1966.

Morris RJ. *Cholera, 1832: The Social Response to an Epidemic*. London: Croom Helm, 1976.

Richardson BW. 'The Life of John Snow', in: Snow J. *On Chloroform and Other Anaesthetics*. London: Churchill, 1858.

Vinten-Johansen P, Brody H, Paneth N, Rachman S, Rip M. *Cholera, Chloroform and the Science of Medicine*. OUP, 2003.

INTRODUCTION

Frazer, James. *Narrative of a Journey into Khorasan*. London: Longman, Hurst, Rees, 1825.

Kennedy, James. *History of the Contagious Cholera*. London: Cochrane, 1831.

Macnamara, C. *A History of Asiatic Cholera*. London: Macmillan, 1876.

Macpherson, John. 'On the Early Seats of Cholera in India and in the East'. In: *Transactions of the Epidemiological Society of London*. Vol 111: 1866–1875. London: T. Richards, 1876.

Scott, William. Report on the Epidemic Cholera. Edinburgh: William Blackwood, 1849.

Smith, Ashbel. *The Cholera Spasmodica, as Observed in Paris in 1832*. New York: P. Hill, 1832.

Sutherland, Robert. 'On the Epidemic of Cholera in the Punjab, the North-West and Central Provinces'. In: *Transactions of the Epidemiological Society of London*. Vol. 111: 1866–1875. London: T. Richards, 1876.

Sydenham, Thomas. *Dr Sydenham's Compleat Method of Curing Almost All Diseases, and Description of their Symptoms*. London: Motte and Bathurst, 1737.

CHAPTER 1

Board of Health minutes and correspondence: PRO/PC/1/101; PC/1/105; PC/1/4395.

Durey M. *The Return of the Plague*. Dublin: Gill and Macmillan, 1979.

McGrew R. *Russia and the Cholera, 1823–1832'*. Madison: University of Wisconsin Press, 1965.

CHAPTER 2

Board of Health minutes and correspondence: PRO/PC/1/101; PC/1/105; PC/1/4395.

Blane, G. *Select Dissertations on Several Subjects of Medical Science*. London: Thomas and George Underwood, 1822.

Bynum WF. *Science and the Practice of Medicine in the Nineteenth Century*. Cambridge: Cambridge University Press, 1994.

Forbes J, Tweedie A, Conolly J (eds). *The Cyclopædia of Practical Medicine*. London: Sherwood, Gilbert and Piper, 1833–1835.

Loudon, ISL. *Medical Care and the General Practitioner, 1750–1858*. Oxford: Clarenden Press, 1986.

Morris R, Kenrick J. *The Edinburgh Medical and Physical Dictionary*. Edinburgh: Bell and Bradfute, 1807.

Paget S (ed). *Memoirs and Letters of Sir James Paget*. London: Longmans, Green, 1903.

Pearce, Evelyn. *Medical and Nursing Dictionary*. London: Faber & Faber, 1941.

Richardson BW. *Vita Medica*. London: Longmans, Green, 1897.

CHAPTER 3

Clanny, William Reid. *Hyperanthraxis or the Cholera of Sunderland*. London: Whittaker, 1832.

Haslewood W, Mordey W. *History and Medical Treatment of Cholera, as it Appeared in Sunderland in 1831*. London: Longman, 1832.

Home Office papers: HO/44/49; HO/31/17.

Kell, James Butler. *On the Appearance of Cholera at Sunderland in 1831*. Edinburgh: Adam and Charles Black, 1834.

The Sunderland Herald.

CHAPTER 4

Board of Health papers PRO/PC1/114; PC1/102.

Chamberlaine, William. *Tirocinium medicum*; Or a dissertation on the duties of youth apprenticed to the medical profession. London: Chamberlaine, 1812.

Cole, Hubert. *Things for the Surgeon: A History of the Resurrection.* London: Heinemann, 1964.

Evidence to the Select Committee Appointed to Inquire into the Manner of Obtaining Subjects for Dissection in the Schools of Anatomy. April 1828. Guildhall Library ref: 1828 vol. V11.1.

Galbraith S. *Dr John Snow: His early years.* London: Royal Institute of Public Health, 2002.

Greville, Charles. *The Greville Memoirs: A Journal of the Reigns of King George IV and King William IV.* (Ed: Henry Reeve). London: Longmans, Green, 1875.

Molison, Thomas. *Remarks on the Epidemic Disease Called Cholera as it Occurred in Newcastle in 1832.* Edinburgh: McLachlan & Stewart, 1832.

Newton, John Frank. *The Return to Nature or Defence of the Vegetable Regimen.* London: 1822.

Shapter, Thomas. *The History of the Cholera in Exeter in 1832.* London: J. Churchill, 1849.

Snow, Stephanie. 'John Snow MD: A Yorkshire childhood and family life'. *Journal of Medical Biography* 2000; 8: 1.

Winskill, P. The Temperance Movement and its Workers. Vol 1. London: Blackie, 1892.

Wright, Thomas Giordani. *Diary of a Doctor: Surgeon's Assistant in Newcastle 1826–1829* (Ed: Alastair Johnson). Newcastle upon Tyne: Newcastle Libraries/Tyne & Wear Archives, 1998.

CHAPTER 5

Erichson, Hugo. *The London Medical Student and Other Comicalities.* Detroit: Detroit Free Press, 1885.

Halford, Henry. *On the Education and Conduct of a Physician.* London: J. Murray, 1834.

Humble JG, Hansell P. *Westminster Hospital, 1716–1966.* London: Pitman Medical, 1966.

Langdon-Davies, John. *Westminster Hospital: Two Centuries of Voluntary Service, 1719–1948.* London: Murray, 1952.

Loudon, ISL. *Medical Care and the General Practitioner, 1750–1858.* Oxford: Clarendon Press, 1986.

Paget S (ed). *Memoirs and Letters of Sir James Paget.* London: Longmans, Green, 1903.

Peterson, M. Jeanne. *The Medical Profession in Mid-Victorian London.* Berkeley: University of California Press, 1978.

Snow, John. *On the Inhalation of the Vapour of Ether in Surgical Operations.* London: Wilson & Ogilvy, 1847.

Snow, Stephanie. 'John Snow MD: Becoming a doctor'. *Journal of Medical Biography* 2000; 8: 2.

CHAPTER 6

Ellis R (ed). *The Case Books of Dr. John Snow.* London: Wellcome Institute for the History of Medicine, 1994.

Simpson, Eve Blantyre. *Sir James Y. Simpson.* Edinburgh: Oliphant, Anderson & Ferrier, 1896.

CHAPTER 7

Board of Health minutes, November 1848 to August 1849.

Edinburgh Medical and Surgical Journal. 1849: 71.

The *Examiner*, various dates, 1849.

Finer, SE. *The Life and Times of Sir Edwin Chadwick.* London: Methuen, 1952.

Poor Law Commissioners. Inquiry into the Sanitary Condition of the Labouring Population of Great Britain. London: HMSO, 1842.

Wohl AS. *Endangered Lives: Public Health in Victorian Britain.* London: Methuen, 1984.

CHAPTER 8

General Board of Health. Report on the Epidemic Cholera of 1848–49. HMSO: London, 1850.

The *London Gazette*. Sept 18th, 1849.

Parkes, E. *British and Foreign Medico-chirurgical Review 1855*; 15: 449–463.

Snow, John. *On the Mode of Communication of Cholera.* London: John Churchill, 1849.

CHAPTER 9

Aristotle. *Historia Animalium.* (Trans.: A.L. Peck) London: Heinemann, 1965.

Bassi Agostino. *Del Mal del Segno* (Trans.: Yarrow PJ). Baltimore: American Phytopathological Society, 1958.

Boyer P, Nissenbaum S (eds). The Salem Witchcraft Papers. Verbatim transcripts of the legal documents of the Salem witchcraft outbreak of 1692. Electronic Text Center, University of Virginia Library.

Brock TD. *Milestones in Microbiology: 1546 to 1940*. Washington, DC: ASM Press, 1999.

Carozzi M. Bonnet, Spallanzani, and Voltaire on regeneration of heads in snails. *Gesnerus 1985*; 42, 3/4.

Cowdell C. *A Disquisition on Pestilential Cholera*. London: Highley, 1848.

Fracastoro G. *De Contagione et Contagiosis Morbis et Eorum Curatione*. (Trans.: Wright WC). New York: Putnam, 1930.

Leeuwenhoek, Antoni van. *The Select Works* (Trans.: Hoole S). London: Hoole, 1799.

Major RH. 'Agostino Bassi and the parasitic theory of disease'. *Bulletin of the History of Medicine* 1944; vol. 16.

Marten B. *A New Theory of Consumptions*. London: Knaplock, Bell, Hooke and King, 1720.

Matossian MK. *Poisons of the Past*. New Haven: Yale University Press, 1989.

Mitchell JK. *On the Crytogamous Origin of Malarious and Epidemic Fevers*. Philadelphia: Lea and Blanchard, 1849.

Needham JT. *An Account of Some New Microscopical Discoveries*. London: Needham, 1745.

Redi, Francesco. *Experiments on the Generation of Insects*. (Trans.: Bigelow, M). Chicago: Open Court, 1909.

Ruestow EG. 'Leeuwenhoek and the Campaign against Spontaneous Generation'. *Journal of the History of Biology 1984*; 17.

Sennert D, Cole A, Culpepper N. *Thirteen Books of Natural Philosophy*. London: P. Cole, 1660.

Wainwright M. *Microbiology before Pasteur*. *Microbiology Today* 2001; 28.

Waller J. *The Discovery of the Germ*. Cambridge: Icon, 2002.

Youngson AJ. *The Scientific Revolution in Victorian Medicine*. London: Croom Helm, 1979.

CHAPTER 10

Adams F. *The Genuine Works of Hippocrates*. Baltimore: Williams & Wilkins, 1939.

Aristotle. *Historia Animalium*. (Trans.: A.L. Peck) London: Heinemann, 1965.

Baly W, Gull W. *Reports on Epidemic Cholera*. London: Royal College of Physicians, 1853.

Bassi Agostino. *Del Mal del Segno* (Trans.: Yarrow PJ). Baltimore: American Phytopathological Society, 1958.

Board of Health minute books, 1848–1854: PRO/MH/5/1–5/12.

Boyer P, Nissenbaum S (eds). The Salem Witchcraft Papers. Verbatim transcripts of the legal documents of the Salem witchcraft outbreak of 1692. Electronic Text Center, University of Virginia Library.

Brock TD. *Milestones in Microbiology: 1546 to 1940*. Washington, DC: ASM Press, 1999.

Carozzi M. Bonnet, Spallanzani, and Voltaire on regeneration of heads in snails. *Gesnerus 1985*; 42, 3/4.

Cowdell C. *A Disquisition on Pestilential Cholera*. London: Highley, 1848.

Fracastoro G. *De Contagione et Contagiosis Morbis et Eorum Curatione*. (Trans.: Wright WC). New York: Putnam, 1930.

Gortvay G, Zoltán I. *Semmelweis: His Life and Work*. Budapest: Akademiai Kiadó, 1968.

Leeuwenhoek, Antoni van. *The Select Works* (Trans.: Hoole S). London: Hoole, 1799.

Pelling M. *Cholera, Fever and English Medicine, 1825–1865*. Oxford: OUP, 1978.

Rockett I. *Population and Health: An Introduction to Epidemiology*. Washington, DC: Population Reference Bureau, 1994.

CHAPTER 11

General Board of Health. Report of the Committee for Scientific Inquiries in Relation to the Cholera Epidemic of 1854. London: HMSO, 1855.

Haldane E. *Mrs Gaskell and Her Friends*. London: Hodder and Stoughton, 1930.

Lockie A, Geddes N. *The Complete Guide to Homeopathy*. London: Dorling Kindersley, 2001.

Woodham-Smith, CB. *Florence Nightingale, 1820–1910*. Harmondsworth, Middlesex: Penquin Books, 1955.

CHAPTER 12

Correspondence: Sir Benjamin Hall and Lord Palmerston, August 1854. University of Southampton library.

Finer SE. *The Life and Times of Sir Edwin Chadwick*. London: Methuen, 1980.

Hassall AH. *Food and its Adulterations: Comprising the Reports of the*

Analytical Sanitary Commission of 'The Lancet' for the Years 1851 to 1854. London: Longman, 1855.

Marion F. *Wonderful Balloon Ascents: Or the Conquest of the Skies*. London: Cassell, Petter & Galpin, 1874.

Parliamentary Papers, July 6th and 31st, 1854.

Snow, J. 'On the adulteration of bread as a cause of rickets'. The *Lancet* 1857; ii: 4–5.

CHAPTER 13

Board of Health minutes, 14th June–1st Nov 1854. MH/5/10.

Board of Health minutes. PRO/MH13/245.

The Builder, September 9th 1854; October 20th, 1855.

CHAPTER 15

Chave, SPW. 'Henry Whitehead and Cholera in Broad Street'. *Medical History 1958*; 2.

Cholera Inquiry Committee. 'Report of the Cholera Outbreak in the Parish of St. James, Westminster during the Autumn of 1854'. London: 1855.

English, Mary. *Victorian Values: The Life and Times of Dr Edwin Lankester*. London: Biopress, 1990.

General Board of Health/John Simon. Report on the Last Two Cholera-Epidemics of London, as Affected by the Consumption of Impure Water. London: HMSO, 1856.

General Board of Health. Report of the Committee for Scientific Inquiries in Relation to the Cholera Epidemic of 1854. London: HMSO, 1855.

Rawnsley HD. *Henry Whitehead: A Memorial Sketch*. Glasgow: James Maclehose, 1898.

Snow, J. *On the Mode of Communication of Cholera* (2nd ed). London: John Churchill, 1855.

Vestry of St James's Westminster, Minutes, 2nd November, 1854 (MSS Westminster City Archives).

Whitehead H. *The Cholera in Berwick Street*. London, 1854.

CHAPTER 16

Eyler, J. *Victorian Social Medicine: The Ideas and Methods of William Farr*. Baltimore: John Hopkins University Press, 1979.

Halliday S. *The Great Stink of London*. Stroud: Sutton, 1999.

Ninth Annual Report of the Medical Officer of the Privy Council. Parliamentary Papers 1867, vol xxxvii.

Parliamentary Papers 1868, vol xxxviii.

Report on the Cholera Epidemics of 1866 in England – Supplement to the 29th annual Report of the Registrar-General of Births, Deaths and Marriages in England. London: HMSO 1867.

Sack D, Sack RB, Nair GB, Siddique AK. 'Cholera'. *Lancet* 2004; 363: 223–33.

Stevens W. *Observations on the Nature and Treatment of the Asiatic Cholera*. London; New York: Hippolyte Baillière, 1853.

Warrell DA et al (eds). *Oxford Textbook of Medicine*. Oxford: Oxford University Press, 2003.

EPILOGUE

Budd W. *Typhoid Fever: Its Nature, Mode of Spreading and Prevention*. London: Longmans, Green, 1873.

Hassall AH. *The Narrative of a Busy Life*. London: Longman, 1893.

Lankester E. Cholera: *What It Is and How to Prevent It*. London, 1866.

INDEX

Figures in italics indicate captions. 'JS' indicates John Snow.